Newborn Screening in Japan—2021

Newborn Screening in Japan—2021

Editors

Toshihiro Tajima
Seiji Yamaguchi

MDPI • Basel • Beijing • Wuhan • Barcelona • Belgrade • Manchester • Tokyo • Cluj • Tianjin

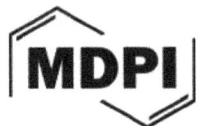

Editors
Toshihiro Tajima
Jichi Children's
Medical Center Tochigi
Japan

Seiji Yamaguchi
Shimane University
School of Medicine
Japan

Editorial Office
MDPI
St. Alban-Anlage 66
4052 Basel, Switzerland

This is a reprint of articles from the Topical Collection published online in the open access journal *International Journal of Neonatal Screening* (ISSN 2409-515X) (available at: https://www.mdpi.com/journal/IJNS/special_issues/japan).

For citation purposes, cite each article independently as indicated on the article page online and as indicated below:

LastName, A.A.; LastName, B.B.; LastName, C.C. Article Title. *Journal Name* **Year**, *Volume Number*, Page Range.

ISBN 978-3-0365-2924-0 (Hbk)
ISBN 978-3-0365-2925-7 (PDF)

© 2022 by the authors. Articles in this book are Open Access and distributed under the Creative Commons Attribution (CC BY) license, which allows users to download, copy and build upon published articles, as long as the author and publisher are properly credited, which ensures maximum dissemination and a wider impact of our publications.

The book as a whole is distributed by MDPI under the terms and conditions of the Creative Commons license CC BY-NC-ND.

Contents

About the Editors vii

Toshihiro Tajima
Newborn Screening in Japan—2021
Reprinted from: *Int. J. Neonatal Screen.* 2022, 8, 3, doi:10.3390/ijns8010003 1

Kenji Yamada, Kazunori Yokoyama, Kikumaro Aoki, Takeshi Taketani and Seiji Yamaguchi
Long-Term Outcomes of Adult Patients with Homocystinuria before and after Newborn Screening
Reprinted from: *Int. J. Neonatal Screen.* 2020, 6, 60, doi:10.3390/ijns6030060 5

Kenji Yamada, Seiji Yamaguchi, Kazunori Yokoyama, Kikumaro Aoki and Takeshi Taketani
Long-Term Neurological Outcomes of Adult Patients with Phenylketonuria before and after Newborn Screening in Japan
Reprinted from: *Int. J. Neonatal Screen.* 2021, 7, 21, doi:10.3390/ijns7020021 13

Shino Odagiri, Daijiro Kabata, Shogo Tomita, Satoshi Kudo, Tomoko Sakaguchi, Noriko Nakano, Kouji Yamamoto, Haruo Shintaku and Takashi Hamazaki
Clinical and Genetic Characteristics of Patients with Mild Hyperphenylalaninemia Identified by Newborn Screening Program in Japan
Reprinted from: *Int. J. Neonatal Screen.* 2021, 7, 17, doi:10.3390/ijns7010017 23

Kanshi Minamitani
Newborn Screening for Congenital Hypothyroidism in Japan
Reprinted from: *Int. J. Neonatal Screen.* 2021, 7, 34, doi:10.3390/ijns7030034 33

Keisuke Nagasaki, Hidetoshi Sato, Sunao Sasaki, Hiromi Nyuzuki, Nao Shibata, Kentaro Sawano, Shota Hiroshima and Tadashi Asami
Re-Evaluation of the Prevalence of Permanent Congenital Hypothyroidism in Niigata, Japan: A Retrospective Study
Reprinted from: *Int. J. Neonatal Screen.* 2021, 7, 27, doi:10.3390/ijns7020027 41

Atsumi Tsuji-Hosokawa and Kenichi Kashimada
Thirty-Year Lessons from the Newborn Screening for Congenital Adrenal Hyperplasia (CAH) in Japan
Reprinted from: *Int. J. Neonatal Screen.* 2021, 7, 36, doi:10.3390/ijns7030036 47

Yosuke Shigematsu, Miori Yuasa, Nobuyuki Ishige, Hideki Nakajima and Go Tajima
Development of Second-Tier Liquid Chromatography-Tandem Mass Spectrometry Analysis for Expanded Newborn Screening in Japan
Reprinted from: *Int. J. Neonatal Screen.* 2021, 7, 44, doi:10.3390/ijns7030044 63

Go Tajima, Reiko Kagawa, Fumiaki Sakura, Akari Nakamura-Utsunomiya, Keiichi Hara, Miori Yuasa, Yuki Hasegawa, Hideo Sasai and Satoshi Okada
Current Perspectives on Neonatal Screening for Propionic Acidemia in Japan: An Unexpectedly High Incidence of Patients with Mild Disease Caused by a Common *PCCB* Variant
Reprinted from: *Int. J. Neonatal Screen.* 2021, 7, 35, doi:10.3390/ijns7030035 77

Reiko Kagawa, Go Tajima, Takako Maeda, Fumiaki Sakura, Akari Nakamura-Utsunomiya, Keiichi Hara, Yutaka Nishimura, Miori Yuasa, Yosuke Shigematsu, Hiromi Tanaka, Saki Fujihara, Chiyoko Yoshii and Satoshi Okada
Pilot Study on Neonatal Screening for Methylmalonic Acidemia Caused by Defects in the Adenosylcobalamin Synthesis Pathway and Homocystinuria Caused by Defects in Homocysteine Remethylation
Reprinted from: *Int. J. Neonatal Screen.* **2021**, 7, 39, doi:10.3390/ijns7030039 85

Tomokazu Kimizu, Shinobu Ida, Kentaro Okamoto, Hiroyuki Awano, Emma Tabe Eko Niba, Yogik Onky Silvana Wijaya, Shin Okazaki, Hideki Shimomura, Tomoko Lee, Koji Tominaga, Shin Nabatame, Toshio Saito, Takashi Hamazaki, Norio Sakai, Kayoko Saito, Haruo Shintaku, Kandai Nozu, Yasuhiro Takeshima, Kazumoto Iijima, Hisahide Nishio and Masakazu Shinohara
Spinal Muscular Atrophy: Diagnosis, Incidence, and Newborn Screening in Japan
Reprinted from: *Int. J. Neonatal Screen.* **2021**, 7, 45, doi:10.3390/ijns7030045 95

About the Editors

Toshihiro Tajima is a professor at Jichi Medical University Children's Medical Center Tochigi. He studied pediatric endocrine diseases at Hokkaido University, Tohoku University, Jichi Medical University and the National Institutes of Health in the USA. He is engaged in the study of congenital hypothyroidism and congenital adrenal hyperplasia found in newborn screening, and has developed guidelines for these diseases in Japan.

Seiji Yamaguchi is a professor at Shimane University's Department of Pediatrics and the former President of the Japanese Society for Neonatal Screening. He has mainly studied organic acidemias and fatty acid oxidation defects, and has contributed as a principal investigator of government project grants to expand newborn screening, introducing tandem mass spectrometry in Japan.

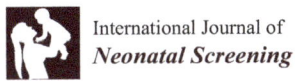

Editorial

Newborn Screening in Japan—2021

Toshihiro Tajima

Jichi Children's Medical Center Tochigi, Jichi Medical University, Shimotsuke-shi 329-0498, Japan; t-tajima@jichi.ac.jp

Japan's Newborn Mass Screening (NBS) was started in 1977 for amino acid metabolism disorders (phenylketonuria (PKU), homocystinuria, maple syrup urine, histidineemia (discontinued in 1993)) and galactosemia at the national level as a national project. Subsequently, congenital hypothyroidism was added in 1979, congenital adrenal hyperplasia was added in 1989, and screening was being conducted for six diseases.

From 2014, a tandem mass analyzer (tandem mass) was introduced nationwide in place of the conventional Guthrie test, and in addition to the conventional amino acid metabolism disorders, urea cycle disorders, organic acid metabolism disorders and fatty acid metabolism disorders have joined the target diseases. Screening is currently being conducted for 20 diseases. The acceptance rate of mass screening in Japan is 100%, and the world's top-level screening, such as quality control system and inspection system, is being carried out.

The Japanese Society for Neonatal Screening was established in 1973 and is now a subcommittee of the Japan Pediatric Society. Members are composed of clinicians (pediatrics, obstetrics and gynecology, internal medicine, etc.), laboratory technicians, basic medical researchers, public health/epidemiological researchers, and administrative personnel.

At this time, the past, present and future of mass screening in Japan is summarized in the Topical Collection of the *International Journal of Neonatal Screening*. I would like to thank everyone involved.

This Topical Collection includes the following topics that are important in newborn screening:

- Long-term prognosis of congenital metabolic diseases found by newborn screening
- Screening issues for congenital hypothyroidism and congenital adrenal hyperplasia
- Challenges of tandem mass screening and new knowledge in Japan
- Screening for spinal muscular atrophy (SMA)

Examination of the long-term prognosis of the diseases found in NBS is an important point. Yamada et al. have investigated the prognosis of adult patients with homocystinuria (HCU) [1] and phenylketonuria (PKU) [2]. HCU revealed that cases found by NBS had a generally good neurological prognosis and general social life. However, it was suggested that Marfanoid and psychiatric symptoms may worsen with age even with treatment. In PKU, pre-NBS patients had some neurological complications, but many patients found by NBS lived a normal social life without neurological problems. However, even patients found with NBS had neuropsychiatric complications in those who discontinued treatment.

It is known that there are many carriers of the PAH gene c.158G> A (p.R53H) in East Asia. Hyperpheylalaninemia (HPA) was also found in the NBS of PKU, but its follow-up policy is not clear in some parts. Odagiri et al. [3] analyzed the genotype and phenotype of Japanese PKU and HPA patients in a large number of cases. As a result, HPA carrying a variant of p.R53H was untreated, and its Phe level was below 360 μmol/L. Therefore, they propose a follow-up method of HPA.

Congenital hypothyroidism (CH) is the most common disease found by NBS. Minamitani [4] discusses changes in the TSH cut-off of CH screening in Japan, an overview of guidelines for CH diagnosis and treatment, screening for low-birth-weight infants and an increase in the frequency of CH in Japan, as in the rest of the world. Furthermore, Nagasaki et al. [5] follow up with patients with CH found in NBS up to the age of 15 and re-evaluate during that course to examine the frequency of permanent CH and transient CH. As a result, it was shown that the frequency of permanent CH is 1 in 2500–3000, which is almost the same as in other countries. Regarding congenital adrenal hyperplasia (CAH), Tsuji-Hosokawa et al. [6] have reported the data of 30 years in the Tokyo Metropolitan area. One of the problems with CAH's NBS is that it has a high false positive rate. Simultaneous measurement of 17-OHP and other steroids has been successful in reducing the false positive rate.

On the topic of tandem screening, Shigematsu et al. [7] have reported in detail the development of a new secondary test method using liquid chromatography-tandem mass spectrometry for the purpose of reducing the false positive rate. Tajima et al. [8] have described the current state of NBS in Japan for Propionic acidemia. The PCCB gene c.1304T> C (p.Y435C) variant is particularly frequently found in Japanese people, so Propionic acidemia is found in 1 in 45,000 people. The cases harboring this variant are considered to be mild, but the treatment and follow-up policy has not yet been determined.

Kagawa et al. [9] have reported cases of cobalamin disorders and methylenetetrahydrofolate reductase deficiency that cannot be detected by the current tandem mass screening. They are investigating improvements in tandem mass screening to detect these cases.

Nucleic acid drug therapy and gene replacement therapy have been developed for SMA, and NBS has been introduced in other countries. On the other hand, although the introduction to NBS is delayed in Japan, Kimizu [10] et al. have reported the frequency of SMA in Japan and the pilot study of NBS and discussed how to introduce NBS for SMA in Japan.

We would like to thank the authors for providing the cutting-edge article series including NBS achievements, problems, solutions, and new screenings that will be developed in the future in Japan. We would also like to thank the reviewers for carefully reviewing the submitted papers and increasing their scientific value.

We will continue to make efforts so that the Japanese Society for Neonatal Screening can contribute to newborn screening. We look forward to overcoming the COVID-19 pandemic and meeting you at the Scientific Meeting of the International Society for Neonatal Screening.

Funding: This research received no external funding.

Conflicts of Interest: The author declares no conflict of interest.

References

1. Kenji, Y.; Kazunori, Y.; Kikumaro, A.; Takeshi, T.; Seiji, Y. Long-Term Outcomes of Adult Patients with Homocystinuria before and after Newborn Screening. *Int. J. Neonatal Screen* **2020**, *6*, 60. [CrossRef]
2. Kenji, Y.; Seiji, Y.; Kazunori, Y.; Kikumaro, A.; Takeshi, T. Long-Term Neurological Outcomes of Adult Patients with Phenylketonuria before and after Newborn Screening in Japan. *Int. J. Neonatal Screen* **2021**, *7*, 21. [CrossRef]
3. Shino, O.; Daijiro, K.; Shogo, T.; Satoshi, K.; Tomoko, S.; Noriko, N.; Kouji, Y.; Haruo, S.; Takashi, H. Clinical and Genetic Characteristics of Patients with Mild Hyperphenylalaninemia Identified by Newborn Screening Program in Japan. *Int. J. Neonatal Screen* **2021**, *7*, 17. [CrossRef]
4. Kanshi, M. Newborn Screening for Congenital Hypothyroidism in Japan. *Int. J. Neonatal Screen* **2021**, *7*, 34. [CrossRef]
5. Keisuke, N.; Hidetoshi, S.; Sunao, S.; Hiromi, N.; Nao, S.; Kentaro, S.; Shota, H.; Tadashi, A. Re-Evaluation of the Prevalence of Permanent Congenital Hypothyroidism in Niigata, Japan: A Retrospective Study. *Int. J. Neonatal Screen* **2021**, *7*, 27. [CrossRef]
6. Atsumi, T.-H.; Kenichi, K. Thirty-Year Lessons from the Newborn Screening for Congenital Adrenal Hyperplasia (CAH) in Japan. *Int. J. Neonatal Screen* **2021**, *7*, 36. [CrossRef]
7. Yosuke, S.; Miori, Y.; Nobuyuki, I.; Hideki, N.; Go, T. Development of Second-Tier Liquid Chromatography-Tandem Mass Spectrometry Analysis for Expanded Newborn Screening in Japan. *Int. J. Neonatal Screen* **2021**, *7*, 44. [CrossRef]
8. Go, T.; Reiko, K.; Fumiaki, S.; Akari, N.-U.; Keiichi, H.; Miori, Y.; Yuki, H.; Hideo, S.; Satoshi, O. Current Perspectives on Neonatal Screening for Propionic Acidemia in Japan: An Unexpectedly High Incidence of Patients with Mild Disease Caused by a Common PCCB Variant. *Int. J. Neonatal Screen* **2021**, *7*, 35. [CrossRef]

9. Reiko, K.; Go, T.; Takako, M.; Fumiaki, S.; Akari, N.-U.; Keiichi, H.; Yutaka, N.; Miori, Y.; Yosuke, S.; Hiromi, T.; et al. Pilot Study on Neonatal Screening for Methylmalonic Acidemia Caused by Defects in the Adenosylcobalamin Synthesis Pathway and Homocystinuria Caused by Defects in Homocysteine Remethylation. *Int. J. Neonatal Screen* **2021**, *7*, 39. [CrossRef]
10. Tomokazu, K.; Shinobu, I.; Kentaro, O.; Hiroyuki, A.; Emma TE, N.; Yogik OS, W.; Shin, O.; Hideki, S.; Tomoko Lee Koji, T.; Tominaga, K.; et al. Spinal Muscular Atrophy: Diagnosis, Incidence, and Newborn Screening in Japan. *Int. J. Neonatal Screen* **2021**, *7*, 45. [CrossRef]

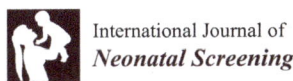

Article

Long-Term Outcomes of Adult Patients with Homocystinuria before and after Newborn Screening

Kenji Yamada [1,*], Kazunori Yokoyama [2], Kikumaro Aoki [2], Takeshi Taketani [1] and Seiji Yamaguchi [1]

1. Department of Pediatrics, Shimane University Faculty of Medicine, 89-1, En-ya-cho, Izumo, Shimane 693-8501, Japan; ttaketani@med.shimane-u.ac.jp (T.T.); seijiyam@med.shimane-u.ac.jp (S.Y.)
2. Secretariat of Special Formula, Aiiku Maternal and Child Health Center, Imperial Gift Foundation Boshi-Aiiku-Kai, 5-6-8, Minami Asabu, Minato-ku, Tokyo 106-8580, Japan; milk@boshiaiikukai.jp (K.Y.); aoki@boshiaiikukai.jp (K.A.)
* Correspondence: k-yamada@med.shimane-u.ac.jp; Tel.: +81-853-20-2219; Fax: +81-853-20-2215

Received: 1 July 2020; Accepted: 29 July 2020; Published: 30 July 2020

Abstract: Background: Homocystinuria (HCU) is a rare inherited metabolic disease. In Japan, newborn screening (NBS) for HCU (cystathionine β-synthase deficiency) was initiated in 1977. We compared the outcomes between patients detected by NBS (NBS group) and clinically detected patients (non-NBS group). Methods: We administered questionnaires about clinical symptoms and social conditions to 16 attending physicians of 19 adult HCU patients treated with methionine-free formula. Results: Eighteen patients (nine patients each in the NBS and non-NBS groups) participated. The frequency of patients with ocular, vascular, central nervous system, and skeletal symptoms in the NBS group was lower than that in the non-NBS group. Intellectual disability was observed in one and eight patients in the NBS and non-NBS groups, respectively. Concerning their social conditions, all patients in the NBS group were employed or still attending school, while only two patients in the non-NBS group were employed. Three of the four patients who discontinued treatment presented some symptoms, even in the NBS group. Conclusion: The social and intellectual outcomes of adult Japanese patients with HCU detected by NBS were favorable. However, even in the patients in the NBS group, some symptoms might not be preventable without continuous treatment.

Keywords: homocystinuria; cystathionine β-synthase deficiency; newborn screening; long-term outcome; social outcome; vitamin B_6; methionine

1. Introduction

Homocystinuria (HCU) is a rare inherited metabolic disease characterized by the accumulation of homocysteine (Hcy) and its metabolites in the blood and urine [1,2]. HCU is classically categorized into three types depending on the specific enzymes involved in the metabolism of sulfur-containing amino acids that are deficient. The three types are as follows: (1) cystathionine β-synthase (CBS) deficiency (OMIM, 236200); (2) defect in cobalamin metabolism; (3) methylenetetrahydrofolate reductase deficiency. In CBS deficiency, the conversion of Hcy to cystathionine is impaired, and CBS deficiency is known as classic homocystinuria or homocystinuria type I [3]. The major clinical manifestations of CBS deficiency include the dislocation of the optic lenses, osteoporosis, "marfanoid" habitus, learning difficulties, and a predisposition to thromboembolism [4]. Because CBS deficiency is clinically heterogeneous and exhibits a wide range of outcomes, some patients have severe clinical phenotypes from childhood, while other patients may be asymptomatic until adulthood. Furthermore, CBS deficiency is classified into two phenotypes depending on vitamin B_6 responsiveness. The B_6-responsive type generally results in a milder phenotype [5].

Newborn screening (NBS) for HCU is performed in several countries and regions, including Western Europe, Australia, the United States of America, and Japan [6]. The prevalence varies widely by ethnicity and has been previously reported to range from 1:1800 to 1:1,000,000, with an overall estimated prevalence of 1:344,000 [7–11]. However, the true frequency is unknown and is thought to be higher than the prevalence detected by both NBS and clinical identification [9,12].

In Japan, NBS for HCU was initiated in 1977 and involves measuring methionine (Met) levels as the diagnostic marker. This strategy detects only CBS deficiency. The detection incidence of HCU (CBS deficiency) in Japan has been reported to be 1:800,000 to 1,000,000 births [13]. Early detection by NBS enables therapeutic intervention from early infancy and the maintenance of lower levels of blood Hcy, which may prevent the development of complications and consequently improve clinical outcomes in terms of both mortality and morbidity [14,15]. Although we reported the outcomes of inborn errors of metabolism in Japanese patients, including HCU detected by NBS, fifteen years ago [16], to date, the long-term outcomes of HCU are unknown. Here, we investigated the long-term outcomes in adult HCU patients, including clinically detected cases.

2. Materials and Methods

We sent questionnaires to 16 attending physicians of 19 adult patients with HCU who were older than 20 years as of October 2017 and who continued to be treated with a Met-free amino acid formula supplied by the Secretariat of Special Formula, Aiiku Maternal and Child Health Center. Patients with HCU types 2 and 3 were excluded from this study.

The questionnaires included questions regarding age, sex, clinical form, physical growth, prior NBS, onset age, first symptoms, metabolic data (i.e., blood methionine and Hcy levels), enzyme activity, genotype, treatments, symptoms (i.e., ocular involvement, vascular symptoms, central nervous system (CNS) disorders, and skeletal malformations), degree of intellectual disability, intermittent use of treatments, educational status, working status, marital status, and additional details. In this study, "marfanoid" included only skeletal symptoms, such as excessive height and/or arachnodactyly.

The subjects were divided into two groups, based on whether they underwent NBS as follows: (1) the NBS group was defined as those who underwent NBS after the initiation of NBS in Japan in 1977; (2) the non-NBS group included those who were born before 1977 or who were born in or after 1977 but did not undergo NBS. The results of the non-NBS group were compared with those of the NBS group; no statistical analysis was performed because of the small sample size in this study.

This study was approved by the Institutional Review Board of Shimane University in 28 September 2017 (#20170726-3).

3. Results

We received answers from 18 of 19 adult patients with HCU (response rate of approximately 95%). Ten males and eight females were included. Although 10 patients underwent NBS, one of these patients failed to be diagnosed with HCU based on NBS, and the diagnosis was made after the onset of symptoms. She was included in the non-NBS group. Eventually, the numbers of patients in the NBS and non-NBS groups were the same (9 per group).

3.1. Profiles of the Patients: Biochemical Findings and Treatments

The patient profiles are summarized in Table 1. The male/female ratio was 7/2 in the NBS group and 3/6 in the non-NBS group. The median ages were 25.8 years (21.3–36.7) and 44.3 years (32.2–59.2) in the NBS and non-NBS groups, respectively. Regarding vitamin B_6 responsiveness, six and five patients in the NBS and non-NBS groups were non-B_6 responsive, respectively. Elevated Met was found in a diagnostic test in 12 patients (NBS, eight patients; non-NBS, four patients) with available data. The median Met levels were 1264 μM (456 to 2433) and 565 μM (366 to 3903) in the NBS and non-NBS groups, respectively. Among the nine patients (NBS, five patients; non-NBS, four patients) with available data, the median blood Hcy levels were 71.7 µM (9.1 to 286) and 63.6 µM (22.2 to 292) in the NBS and non-NBS groups, respectively.

Table 1. Overview of the participating Japanese patients with HCU.

	NBS Group ($n = 9$)	Non-NBS Group ($n = 9$)
Sex		
Male	7	3
Female	2	6
Median age (range) (years)	25.8 (21.3–36.7)	44.3 (32.2–59.2)
Clinical form		
B_6 responsive	2	0
Non-B_6 responsive	6	5
Unknown	1	4
Diagnostic test		
Median Met (range) (µM)	1264 ($n = 8$) (456–2433)	565 ($n = 4$) (366–3903)
Median Hcy (range) (µM)	71.7 ($n = 5$) (9.1–286)	63.6 ($n = 4$) (22.2–292)
Number of patients undergoing tests for the urinary excretion of homocystine	7	5
Number of patients undergoing tests for CBS activity	2	2
Number of patients undergoing genetic tests	5	2
Treatments		
Met-free formula	9	9
Protein-restricted diet	7	4
Betaine	9	3
Aspirin	6	3
Dipyridamole	0	0
Others	3	2
Number of patients with a history of treatment interruption	4	2

Met, methionine; Hcy, homocysteine; CBS, cystathionine β-synthase.

In three of the seven patients who underwent genetic testing, five types of variants—namely, p.H65R, p.G116R, p.G259S, p.M382R, and p.F531Gfs*9—in *CBS*, were identified. Only p.G116R was found in two patients. p.M382R was a novel mutation judged as "causing the disease" based on the Mutation Taster (http://www.mutationtaster.org/) results.

In the NBS group, all nine patients were treated with betaine and dietary therapy with Met-free formula, seven patients followed a protein-restricted diet, and six patients underwent antiplatelet therapy with aspirin. Additionally, three patients were treated with vitamin supplementation or anticoagulant therapy as other treatments. Meanwhile, in the non-NBS group, all nine patients received dietary therapy using a Met-free formula, and four patients followed a protein-restricted diet. Betaine and aspirin were administered to three patients. In the non-NBS group, one patient was treated for hypertension and hyperlipidemia, and another patient received antiplatelet therapy other than aspirin.

In total, four and two patients temporarily discontinued the treatment in the NBS and non-NBS groups, respectively. The reasons included economic problems, insufficient instructions by the physicians, and self-judgment mainly due to fewer subjective symptoms experienced during adulthood, difficulty in visiting distant hospitals, decreased motivation, the need for excessively strict control, and/or the cost of betaine. The discontinuation periods ranged from a few years to approximately ten years.

3.2. Clinical Symptoms

The major clinical symptoms in this survey are shown in Table 2. The NBS group had fewer complications than the non-NBS group. In particular, four of the nine patients in the NBS group were asymptomatic, and all patients were in their 20s.

Table 2. Comparison of the major clinical symptoms in adult patients.

		NBS Group (n = 9)		Non-NBS Group (n = 9)		
	Current Age	20s (n = 5)	30s (n = 4)	30s (n = 4)	40s (n = 3)	50s (n = 2)
Eye	ectopia lentis	0	0	2	2	1
	myopia	0	0	0	1	0
	glaucoma	0	0	0	1	1
	other (retinal detachment)	0	1	0	0	0
Vascular system	coronal	0	0	0	0	0
	pulmonary	1	0	0	1	0
	cerebral	0	1	2	1	0
	other	0	0	0	0	1
Central nervous system	intellectual disability	0	1	2	3	2
	epilepsy	0	0	2	0	1
	psychiatric disability	0	2	1	0	0
	other (dystonia)	0	0	0	0	1
Skeletal system	marfanoid #	0	3	2	3	0
	osteoporosis	0	1	1	1	0
	scoliosis	0	0	2	2	1
	pectus excavatum	0	0	1	0	1
	other	0	0	0	0	0
Other *		0	0	1	2	1
No symptoms		4	0	0	0	0

#: marfanoid involves excessive height and/or arachnodactyly. *: other symptoms included diabetes, arteriosclerosis obliterans, hyperlipidemia, and pneumonia in one patient each. The cumulative total number of patients was counted.

Concerning optic involvement, retinal detachment was noted in one of the nine patients in the NBS group, who was aged 35 years, while among the nine patients in the non-NBS group, ectopia lentis, myopia, and glaucoma were observed in five, one and two patients, respectively.

Regarding vascular system complications, one patient in the NBS group had a thromboembolism in the pulmonary vessels at the age of 26 years, and another patient had cerebrovascular thromboembolic events at the age of 31 years. These two patients had a history of treatment interruption. In the non-NBS group, four patients developed thromboembolism in the period between the age of 6 years and their fourth decade of life, and one of them experienced complications of both cerebrovascular and pulmonary vascular obstructions.

Regarding CNS symptoms, psychiatric disability was noted in two of nine patients in the NBS group. One of these two patients with psychiatric disability also had intellectual disability. In contrast, all nine patients in the non-NBS group had some type of CNS symptoms, such as intellectual disability, epilepsy, psychiatric disability, and/or dystonia. Intellectual disability, including that of a mild degree, was observed in seven patients in the non-NBS group.

Regarding complications of the skeletal system, marfanoid was observed in three patients in the NBS group in their 30s. One patient also had osteoporosis. Meanwhile, all patients in the non-NBS group, except for one patient, presented some skeletal symptoms. Marfanoid, osteoporosis, scoliosis, and pectus excavatum were noted in five, two, five, and two patients, respectively.

Other complications, such as diabetes, arteriosclerosis obliterans, hyperlipidemia, and pneumonia, were noted in one patient each in the non-NBS group.

3.3. Life Outcomes: Intelligence, Education, Employment, and Other Outcomes

The outcomes in this survey are shown in Table 3. Physical development was within the normal range in six and three patients in the NBS and non-NBS groups, respectively. In total, two and four patients had excessive height in the NBS and non-NBS groups, respectively. Other physical findings, such as short stature and obesity, were noted in one and two patients in the NBS and non-NBS groups, respectively.

Table 3. Comparison of clinical and social status.

	NBS Group (n = 9)	Non-NBS Group (n = 9)
Physical development		
Normal	6	3
Excessive height	2	4
Other *	1	2
Intelligence		
Normal	8	1
Borderline	0	3
Mild intellectual disability	1	0
Moderate intellectual disability	0	1
Severe intellectual disability	0	1
Unknown degree of intellectual disability (may be moderate or severe)	0	3
Education status		
University	2	2
Technical school	4	0
High school	1	2
Junior high school	0	0
School for handicapped	1	3
Unknown	1	2
Employment status		
Attending school	1	0
Employed	8	2
Unemployed	0	3
Living in a facility for the handicapped	0	3
Unknown	0	1
Marital status		
Married	2	0
Unmarried or not yet married	5	6
Outcome		
Alive	9	6
Dead	0	3

* Other includes obesity or a short stature.

Regarding intelligence, eight patients showed normal intelligence, and one patient had mild intellectual disability among the nine patients in the NBS group. In contrast, only one of the nine patients in the non-NBS group demonstrated normal development, while three patients showed borderline, and one each had moderate and severe intellectual disability. An unknown degree of intellectual disability (may be moderate or severe) was noted in the other three patients in the non-NBS group.

Regarding education status, the final educational attainment was university, vocational school, high school, and school for the handicapped in two, four, one, and one patients, respectively, in the NBS group. In contrast, in the non-NBS group, the numbers of patients were two, zero, two, and three, respectively.

Regarding other outcomes, including employment and marital status, eight of nine patients in the NBS group were employed, and the other patient was still attending school. In the non-NBS group, two patients were employed, and three patients each were unemployed or living in a facility for the handicapped. Two patients in the NBS group were married, while no patient was married in the non-NBS group. Although all nine patients in the NBS group were alive, three patients in the non-NBS group had already died. The causes of death in these three patients were thalamic hemorrhage, pneumonia, and unknown. No further information regarding the three deceased patients was available.

In the other free description, all attending physicians stated the need for life-long treatment. Additionally, some physicians described the need to support medical expenses, including the treatment cost of betaine, and the necessity for consultation with internal medicine and psychiatry specialists.

4. Discussion

Our study revealed that NBS substantially contributed to the improvement in the long-term outcomes of Japanese patients with HCU but that the symptoms might progress even in patients detected by NBS. All patients in the NBS group worked or attended school, and all had normal mental development, except for one patient. NBS for HCU was previously reported to be an effective and recommended program [17]. The early start of treatment to maintain low levels of Hcy improved the long-term outcomes [18], and our study supports the finding that outcomes in Japanese patients are similar to those in previous reports.

Our results also indicate that lifelong continuous treatment is important to the achievement of improved long-term outcomes. Three of the four patients who discontinued their treatments presented some symptoms, even in the NBS group, while three of the five patients continuing treatments were asymptomatic. However, because information regarding the Hcy levels during the treatment period, including the discontinuation period, was not available in our study, the relationship between the outcomes and treatment interruption could not be fully elucidated.

Additionally, our results suggest that, even if HCU is detected by NBS and is continuously treated, the condition is likely to progress in some cases. In our study, the condition of the patients in their 30s seemed to be more severe than that of the patients in their 20s, even within the same NBS group. This finding might indicate that the management was improved or that their symptoms progressed. Our results also explored the responsiveness to treatments. Because marfanoid and psychiatric disability were observed in some patients in the NBS group, these symptoms might not be completely prevented even by early detection and intervention. However, scoliosis and pectus excavatum might be responsive to early intervention because these symptoms were present only in the non-NBS group. Ectopia lentis and intellectual disability also seemed to be responsive to early treatment.

Regarding vitamin B_6 responsiveness, two of 11 patients could be considered B_6-responders in our study, which is similar to a previous report revealing that 15% of Japanese HCU patients were vitamin B_6 responders (based on a report in a domestic Japanese journal). The Japanese prevalence of B_6 responders was higher than that in Ireland, where 1 in 25 patients was a B_6 responders [18], while a report showed that 231 of 629 patients (36.7%) were vitamin B_6 responders [19]. However, because not all Japanese patients, such as pyridoxine-responsive patients treated without Met-free formula, were included in our study, our results for vitamin B_6 responsiveness might not correctly reflect the true prevalence in Japan.

Concerning the genetic background, it has been suggested that p.G116R might be common among Japanese patients, although genetic testing information was available for only three patients. In the European population, it has been reported that the p.I278T mutation is common and is associated with B_6 responsiveness [9]. Additionally, the p.T191M, p.G307S, and p.R336C mutations are relatively common in some populations [8,20,21]. However, these mutations were not observed in the Japanese patients in our study.

Although 1 in 10 patients born between 1977 and 1997 was a false-negative case in our study, our results could not provide information about the sensitivity and specificity of screening tests using Met levels because of the small sample size. It is well known that the sensitivity and specificity of screening tests using Met levels alone are insufficient [22]. The selection of appropriate markers and setting of accurate cut-off values are future challenges for the NBS for HCU in the Japanese population.

There may be some limitations of our study. For example, patients treated with Met-free formula who could be traced by our institution were recruited for our study. Patients treated with only betaine and vitamin B_6, patients who died before adulthood, and patients who interrupted treatment with Met-free formula during this survey, were not included. Information regarding the three dead patients was insufficient. Because approximately 30,000,000 babies were screened between 1977 and 1997 in Japan (1,200,000 to 1,800,000 births per year), there should, theoretically, be approximately 40 adult patients with HCU, but only 10 patients could be enrolled in our study. Therefore, our results do not correctly reflect the long-term outcomes of all Japanese patients with HCU. Furthermore, because HCU is a progressive disease, the differences in outcomes between the two groups may be associated with, not only NBS, but also age. We did not collect information to estimate the severity of disease except for symptoms; therefore, we could not compare disease severity between the two groups. Nevertheless, we believe that the severity is similar between the two groups because the Met and/or Hcy levels in the NBS group at diagnosis were similar to those in the non-NBS group. Therefore, we could not definitively conclude that the positive outcomes were all due to NBS. However, because there are few reports in which the long-term outcomes of patients with HCU detected by NBS were compared with those of clinically detected patients on the same scale and because the long-term outcomes of Japanese patients are unknown, our results are important for the investigation of the effect of NBS on HCU.

5. Conclusions

The long-term, particularly social and intellectual, outcomes of Japanese adult patients with HCU detected by NBS were favorable compared with those of patients with clinically detected HCU. However, even in the patients in the NBS group, some symptoms might not be preventable, and long-term outcomes may worsen if treatment is interrupted.

Author Contributions: Conceptualization, K.Y. (Kenji Yamada), K.A. and S.Y.; Methodology, K.Y. (Kenji Yamada) and S.Y.; Software, K.Y. (Kenji Yamada) and K.Y. (Kazunori Yokoyama); Validation, K.Y. (Kenji Yamada) and K.Y. (Kazunori Yokoyama); Formal Analysis, K.Y. (Kenji Yamada) and K.Y. (Kazunori Yokoyama); Investigation, K.Y. (Kenji Yamada) and S.Y.; Data Curation, K.Y. (Kenji Yamada) and K.Y. (Kazunori Yokoyama); Writing—Original Draft Preparation, K.Y. (Kenji Yamada); Writing—Review and Editing, K.Y. (Kazunori Yokoyama), K.A., T.T. and S.Y.; Visualization, K.Y. (Kenji Yamada); Supervision, K.A., T.T. and S.Y.; Project Administration, K.A., T.T. and S.Y.; Funding Acquisition, K.Y. (Kenji Yamada). All authors have read and agreed to the published version of the manuscript.

Funding: This report was partially supported by AMED (grant number JP20ek0109482) and JSPS KAKENHI (grant number 19K08300). The authors confirm independence from the sponsors; the content of the article was not influenced by the sponsors.

Acknowledgments: We thank O. Sakamoto at Tohoku University, M. Ishige and E. Ogawa at Nihon University, K. Shimura at Tokyo Metropolitan Children's Medical Center, A. Tsuchiya at Tsuchiya Clinic, S. Soneda at St. Marianna University School of Medicine, N. Shimozawa at Gifu University, Y. Maruo at Shiga University of Medical Science Hospital, A. Nishiyama at Kobe University, E. Naito at Tokushima University, T. Miyake at Ehime University, Y. Watanabe at Kurume University, Y. Indo at Kumamoto University, K. Shiomi at Miyazaki University, M. Gotanda at Gotanda Medical Clinic, Y. Maruyama at Imakiire General Hospital, and T. Inoue at Fukiage Clinic for providing patient information and cooperating during the study.

Conflicts of Interest: The authors declare that there are no conflicts of interest. The funders had no role in the design of the study; in the collection, analyses, or interpretation of data; in the writing of the manuscript, or in the decision to publish the results.

References

1. Carson, N.A.; Neill, D.W. Metabolic abnormalities detected in a survey of mentally backward individuals in Northern Ireland. *Arch. Dis. Child.* **1962**, *37*, 505–513. [CrossRef]
2. Gerritsen, T.; Vaughn, J.G.; Waisman, H.A. The identification of homocystine in the urine. *Biochem. Biophys. Res. Commun.* **1962**, *9*, 493–496. [CrossRef]
3. Mudd, S.H.; Finkelstein, J.D.; Irreverre, F.; Laster, L. Homocystinuria: An enzymatic defect. *Science* **1964**, *143*, 1443–1445. [CrossRef] [PubMed]
4. Morris, A.A.; Kozich, V.; Santra, S.; Andria, G.; Ben-Omran, T.I.; Chakrapani, A.B.; Crushell, E.; Henderson, M.J.; Hochuli, M.; Huemer, M.; et al. Chapman, Guidelines for the diagnosis and management of cystathionine beta-synthase deficiency. *J. Inherit. Metab. Dis.* **2017**, *40*, 49–74. [CrossRef] [PubMed]

5. Sacharow, S.J.; Picker, J.D.; Levy, H.L. Homocystinuria Caused by Cystathionine Beta-Synthase Deficiency. In *GeneReviews®*; Adam, M.P., Ardinger, H.H., Pagon, R.A., Wallace, S.E., Bean, L.J.H., Stephens, K., Amemiya, A., Eds.; University of Washington: Seattle, WA, USA, 2004.
6. Walter, J.H.; Jahnke, N.; Remmington, T. *Newborn Screening for Homocystinuria the Cochrane Database of Systematic Reviews*; John Wiley & Sons, Ltd.: Hoboken, NJ, USA, 2015; p. Cd008840.
7. Zschocke, J.; Kebbewar, M.; Gan-Schreier, H.; Fischer, C.; Fang-Hoffmann, J.; Wilrich, J.; Abdoh, G.; Ben-Omran, T.; Shahbek, N.; Lindner, M.; et al. Molecular neonatal screening for homocystinuria in the Qatari population. *Hum. Mutat.* **2009**, *30*, 1021–1022. [CrossRef] [PubMed]
8. Gan-Schreier, H.; Kebbewar, M.; Fang-Hoffmann, J.; Wilrich, J.; Abdoh, G.; Ben-Omran, T.; Shahbek, N.; Bener, A.; Al Rifai, H.; Al Khal, A.L.; et al. Newborn population screening for classic homocystinuria by determination of total homocysteine from Guthrie cards. *J. Pediatr.* **2010**, *156*, 427–432. [CrossRef] [PubMed]
9. Skovby, F.; Gaustadnes, M.; Mudd, S.H. A revisit to the natural history of homocystinuria due to cystathionine beta-synthase deficiency. *Mol. Genet. Metab.* **2010**, *99*, 1–3. [CrossRef] [PubMed]
10. Naughten, E.R.; Yap, S.; Mayne, P.D. Newborn screening for homocystinuria: Irish and world experience. *Eur. J. Pediatr.* **1998**, *157*, S84–S87. [CrossRef] [PubMed]
11. Linnebank, M.; Homberger, A.; Junker, R.; Nowak-Goettl, U.; Harms, E.; Koch, H.G. High prevalence of the I278T mutation of the human cystathionine beta-synthase detected by a novel screening application. *Thromb. Haemost.* **2001**, *85*, 986–988. [CrossRef] [PubMed]
12. Refsum, H.; Fredriksen, A.; Meyer, K.; Ueland, P.M.; Kase, B.F. Birth prevalence of homocystinuria. *J. Pediatr.* **2004**, *144*, 830–832. [PubMed]
13. Aoki, K. Newborn screening in Japan. *Southeast Asian J. Trop. Med. Public Health* **2003**, *34*, 80.
14. Yap, S.; Boers, G.H.; Wilcken, B.; Wilcken, D.E.; Brenton, D.P.; Lee, P.J.; Walter, J.H.; Howard, P.M.; Naughten, E.R. Vascular outcome in patients with homocystinuria due to cystathionine beta-synthase deficiency treated chronically: A multicenter observational study. *Arterioscler. Thromb. Vasc. Biol.* **2001**, *21*, 2080–2085. [CrossRef] [PubMed]
15. Yap, S.; Rushe, H.; Howard, P.M.; Naughten, E.R. The intellectual abilities of early-treated individuals with pyridoxine-nonresponsive homocystinuria due to cystathionine beta-synthase deficiency. *J. Inherit. Metab. Dis.* **2001**, *24*, 437–447. [CrossRef] [PubMed]
16. Aoki, K. Long term follow-up of patients with inborn errors of metabolism detected by the newborn screening program in Japan. *Southeast Asian J. Trop. Med. Public Health* **2003**, *34*, 19–23. [PubMed]
17. Keller, R.; Chrastina, P.; Pavlikova, M.; Gouveia, S.; Ribes, A.; Kolker, S.; Blom, H.J.; Baumgartner, M.R.; Bartl, J.; Dionisi-Vici, C.; et al. Newborn screening for homocystinurias: Recent recommendations versus current practice. *J. Inherit. Metab. Dis.* **2019**, *42*, 128–139. [CrossRef] [PubMed]
18. Yap, S.; Naughten, E. Homocystinuria due to cystathionine beta-synthase deficiency in Ireland: 25 years' experience of a newborn screened and treated population with reference to clinical outcome and biochemical control. *J. Inherit. Metab. Dis.* **1998**, *21*, 738–747. [CrossRef] [PubMed]
19. Mudd, S.H.; Skovby, F.; Levy, H.L.; Pettigrew, K.D.; Wilcken, B.; Pyeritz, R.E.; Andria, G.; Boers, G.H.; Bromberg, I.L.; Cerone, R.; et al. The natural history of homocystinuria due to cystathionine beta-synthase deficiency. *Am. J. Hum. Genet.* **1985**, *37*, 1–31. [PubMed]
20. Cozar, M.; Urreizti, R.; Vilarinho, L.; Grosso, C.; de Kremer, R.D.; Asteggiano, C.G.; Dalmau, J.; Garcia, A.M.; Vilaseca, M.A.; Grinberg, D.; et al. Identification and functional analyses of CBS alleles in Spanish and Argentinian homocystinuric patients. *Hum. Mutat.* **2011**, *32*, 835–842. [CrossRef] [PubMed]
21. Alcaide, P.; Krijt, J.; Ruiz-Sala, P.; Jesina, P.; Ugarte, M.; Kozich, V.; Merinero, B. Enzymatic diagnosis of homocystinuria by determination of cystathionine-ss-synthase activity in plasma using LC-MS/MS. *Clina Chim. Acta* **2015**, *438*, 261–265. [CrossRef] [PubMed]
22. Huemer, M.; Kožich, V.; Rinaldo, P.; Baumgartner, M.R.; Merinero, B.; Pasquini, E.; Ribes, A.; Blom, H.J. Newborn screening for homocystinurias and methylation disorders: Systematic review and proposed guidelines. *J. Inherit. Metab. Dis.* **2015**, *38*, 1007–1019. [CrossRef] [PubMed]

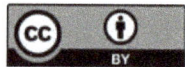

© 2020 by the authors. Licensee MDPI, Basel, Switzerland. This article is an open access article distributed under the terms and conditions of the Creative Commons Attribution (CC BY) license (http://creativecommons.org/licenses/by/4.0/).

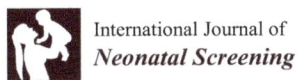

Article

Long-Term Neurological Outcomes of Adult Patients with Phenylketonuria before and after Newborn Screening in Japan

Kenji Yamada [1,*], Seiji Yamaguchi [1], Kazunori Yokoyama [2], Kikumaro Aoki [2] and Takeshi Taketani [1]

1. Department of Pediatrics, Shimane University Faculty of Medicine, 89-1 Enya-cho, Izumo, Shimane 693-8501, Japan; seijiyam@med.shimane-u.ac.jp (S.Y.); ttaketani@med.shimane-u.ac.jp (T.T.)
2. Secretariat of Special Formula, Aiiku Maternal and Child Health Center, Imperial Gift Foundation Boshi-Aiiku-Kai, 5-6-8 Minami Azabu, Minato-ku, Tokyo 106-8580, Japan; milk@boshiaiikukai.jp (K.Y.); aoki@boshiaiikukai.jp (K.A.)
* Correspondence: k-yamada@med.shimane-u.ac.jp; Tel.: +81-853-20-2219; Fax: +81-853-20-2215

Abstract: Japanese newborn screening (NBS) for phenylketonuria (PKU) was initiated in 1977. We surveyed the neurological outcomes of Japanese adult patients with PKU to investigate the long-term effects of and of and issues with NBS. Eighty-five patients with PKU aged over 19 years who continued to be treated with a phenylalanine-free amino acid formula were investigated by administering questionnaires regarding clinical characteristics, such as mental ability, education status, and therapeutic condition. Of the 85 subjects, 68 patients were detected by NBS (NBS group), while the other 17 were clinically diagnosed before the initiation of NBS (pre-NBS group). Further, 10 of the 68 NBS patients presented intellectual and/or psychiatric disabilities, 5 of whom had a history of treatment discontinuation; in contrast, 12 of the 17 pre-NBS patients presented with neuropsychiatric symptoms. Regarding social outcomes, almost all patients in the NBS group could live an independent life, while over half of the patients in the pre-NBS group were not employed or lived in nursing-care facilities. Neurological outcomes are obviously improved by NBS in Japan. However, some patients, even those detected by NBS, developed neuropsychiatric symptoms due to treatment disruption. Lifelong and strict management is essential to maintain good neurological and social prognoses for patients with PKU.

Keywords: phenylketonuria; newborn screening; long-term outcome; adult patients; Japanese; intellectual disability; psychiatric disability; treatment discontinuation

1. Introduction

Phenylketonuria (PKU, OMIM No. 261600), an autosomal recessive inherited disease of amino acid metabolism, is a major disease identified by newborn screening (NBS) [1]. Classic PKU is caused by phenylalanine hydroxylase (PAH, OMIM No. 612349) deficiency and is associated with severe intellectual disability, convulsions, hypopigmentation, behavioral abnormalities, and dementia. Because PKU is detected as an elevation in phenylalanine (Phe) levels in NBS, mild hyperphenylalaninemia (HPA), tetrahydrobiopterin (BH_4) deficiency, including BH_4 metabolic defects, and BH_4-responsive PKU and classic PKU are all detectable. Mild HPA is also caused by a defect in PAH but is clinically mild and may require less strict dietary restrictions. BH_4-responsive PKU and BH_4 deficiency show BH_4 responsiveness. The global prevalence of PKU has been reported to be approximately 1 in 4000 to 15,000 births [1–3], but the incidence of NBS in Japan has been reported to be 1 in 50,000 to 70,000 births [4,5].

NBS for PKU first spread from the mid to late 1960s in North America and the United Kingdom, while nationwide NBS for PKU was initiated in 1977 in Japan. Almost all cases of PKU are detected by NBS and treated immediately after birth. The treatment is mainly a diet with protein restriction and Phe-free formula and supplementation with BH_4 in some cases. With this therapy, the life and neurological prognoses of patients with PKU

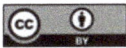

have been reported to improve, at least in childhood, resulting in a significantly decreased societal economic burden [6,7]. Therefore, PKU is considered one of the best targets for NBS in terms of a cost–benefit analysis.

However, even in patients who are initially treated and achieve good metabolic control, reversible (and sometimes irreversible) neuropsychiatric symptoms can develop if this control is lost in later childhood or adulthood [8]. In addition, over time, some patients may manifest subtle intellectual and neuropsychiatric issues even with strict adherence to a low-Phe diet [9–12]. In fact, the long-term outcome of PKU is not necessarily favorable.

In this study, we expanded upon our previous studies [5,13,14] and investigated the social and neurological outcomes of adult patients aged over 20 years who were diagnosed with PKU before and after NBS in Japan using a questionnaire administered to attending doctors.

2. Materials and Methods

We sent questionnaires to the 33 attending physicians of 85 adult patients with PKU aged over 20 years as of October 2016 (born before 1996) who had continuously required a special formula (including Phe-free comprehensive amino acid powder and low-Phe peptide powder) supplied by the Secretariat of Special Formula, Aiiku Maternal and Child Health Center for dietary therapy.

Attending physicians answered the questionnaires based on clinical records. The questionnaire included questions on sex, age, clinical form of PKU, history of treatment interruption and the reason, follow-up department, physical development, neuropsychiatric disability, educational status, work status, and marital status and allowed for an open-ended description of the patient.

Regarding the question on neuropsychiatric disability, attending physicians were able to answer "normal intelligence", "borderline intellectual disability", "intellectual disability", and/or "psychiatric disability". When "intellectual disability" was selected, patients with an IQ (intelligence quotient) less than 50 or patients living in nursing-care facilities were characterized as having a "moderate-severe intellectual disability", while those with an IQ of 50–70 or who are able to fend for themselves and patients with borderline intellectual disability were characterized as having a "borderline-mild intellectual disability". Additionally, the details of psychiatric disability were judged based on the open-ended description. Regarding physical development, short stature was defined as a height <160 cm for males and <148 cm for females. Obesity and leanness were defined as BMI >25 and <18.5 kg/m^2, respectively.

The subjects were divided into the following two groups: (1) the NBS group was defined as patients who underwent NBS, and (2) the pre-NBS group consisted of patients who were born before 1977 (when NBS was initiated) or were born after 1977 but did not receive NBS. Each of the groups was subdivided into age groups of approximately 5 years. The results of the NBS and pre-NBS groups were compared without a statistical analysis because of the small-scale nature of this study.

This study was approved by the Institutional Review Board of Shimane University on 13 October 2016 (#20160915-2).

3. Results

We received answers from the attending physicians of all 85 adult patients with PKU (response rate of 100%). All participants were alive. Because only one patient had not undergone NBS despite being born in 1979, she was enrolled in the pre-NBS group (and classified into the 39–44-year-old subgroup). Eventually, 68 and 17 patients were placed into the NBS and pre-NBS groups, respectively. As shown in Table 1, the NBS group consisted of 34 males and 33 females, while 7 males and 10 females constituted the pre-NBS group. The median age (range) of the NBS and pre-NBS groups was 28.5 years (20.5 to 38.2) and 43.9 years (37.7 to 50.8), respectively. Regarding the clinical form of PKU, almost all patients had classic PKU, but six patients with mild HPA and two patients with BH$_4$-

responsive PKU were included in the NBS group. In this study, almost all participants (66 of the 68 patients in the NBS group and 16 of the 17 patients in the pre-NBS group) were managed by pediatricians even after reaching adulthood.

Table 1. Overview of the participating patients with phenylketonuria (PKU).

		NBS Group (n = 68)	Pre-NBS Group (n = 17)
Sex			
	male	34	7
	female	33	10
	unknown	1	0
Median age (range) [years]		28.5 (20.5–38.2)	43.9 (37.7–50.8)
	20–24	22	0
	25–29	19	0
	30–34	14	0
	35–39	13	3
	40–44	0	7
	45–49	0	6
	50-	0	1
Clinical form			
	classic	54	16
	mild HPA	6	0
	BH$_4$-responsive	2	0
	BH$_4$ defect	0	0
	unknown	6	1
Follow-up department			
	pediatrics	66	16
	internal medicine	1	1
	gynecology	1	0
treatment interruption		21	5

HPA, hyperphenylalaninemia; BH$_4$, tetrahydrobiopterin.

Approximately 30% of patients (21 of the 68 patients in the NBS group and 5 of the 17 patients in the pre-NBS group) had ever discontinued treatment. Although the description of treatment discontinuation was unequal due to the open-ended questionnaire, concrete information was obtained for only eight patients in the NBS group. Among them, the median age at treatment discontinuation was 18 years (range, 11 to 20 years), and the median duration was 11 years (range, a few years to 23 years). In the pre-NBS group, the details of treatment discontinuation were provided by one patient, and she was a 42-year-old female who had several intermittent histories of treatment discontinuation for a total of a few decades beginning at 3 years of age. As shown in Table 2, the most common reasons for discontinuation before and after NBS were financial problems and self-judgment, including a decrease in motivation and busy school or work schedules, followed by the unpleasant taste of the special formula and erroneous recommendations from the attending physicians. On the other hand, the most common reason for restarting dietary therapy is the prevention of maternal PKU, followed by improvement of the medical subsidy system and the appearance of psychiatric or behavioral abnormalities.

Table 2. Reasons for discontinuing or restarting dietary treatment.

Reasons for Discontinuation (Number of Patients with the Same Comment)	Reasons for Restarting (Number of Patients with the Same Comment)
Economic problems (7)	Pregnancy (8)
Self-judgment/personal circumstances (7)	Improvement of the medical subsidy system (4)
Unpleasant taste of the special formula (6)	Appearance of psychiatric abnormalities (3)
Recommendation of the attending physicians (5)	Spontaneously restarted (2)
Changes in one's environment (3)	

Figure 1 shows the comparison of intellectual outcomes before and after NBS in different age groups. Normal intelligence was observed in 60 of the 68 patients (88%) in the NBS group; specifically, all but two patients less than 35 years old had normal intelligence. Meanwhile, even in the NBS group, 6 of 13 patients over 35 years of age exhibited a certain degree of intellectual disability, including 5 patients with borderline intellectual disability. In contrast to the results of the NBS group, only 6 of the 17 patients (35%) in the pre-NBS group showed normal intelligence. Additionally, the degree of intellectual disability in the pre-NBS group was more severe than that in the NBS group.

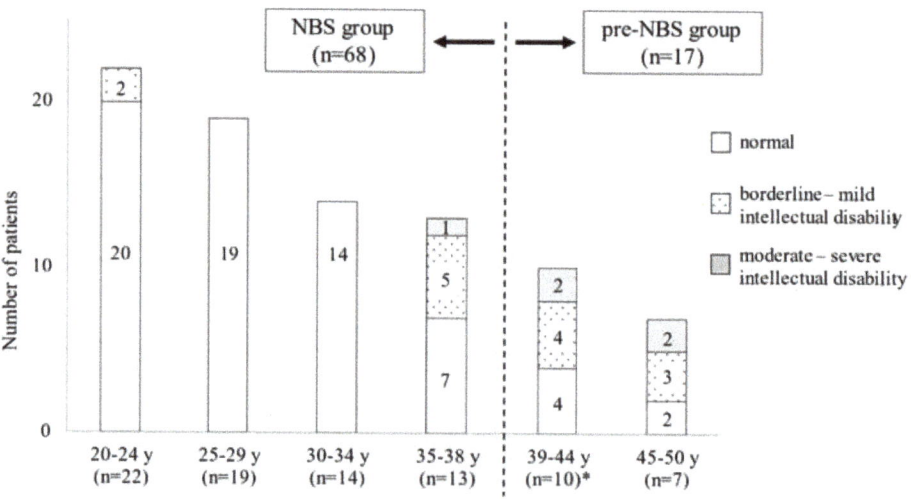

Figure 1. Degree of intellectual disability in patients stratified by age before and after newborn screening.*, A 37-year-old female was included in the "39–44-year-old subgroup" of the pre-newborn screening (NBS) group because she did not undergo NBS.

Table 3 shows a comparison of other clinical symptoms and social outcomes. Regarding the psychiatric status, transient psychiatric disabilities were observed in three patients in the NBS group, all of whom had histories of treatment interruption, during their intermittent treatment. Another patient presented with a psychiatric disability. Four patients presented with an abnormal psychiatric status in the NBS group (6%). On the other hand, 6 of 17 patients (35%) in the pre-NBS group had psychiatric disabilities. When the number of patients with intellectual and/or psychiatric disabilities was counted collectively as neuropsychiatric diseases, the total was 10 patients in the NBS group. More specifically, six patients were diagnosed with only an intellectual disability, two patients were diagnosed with intellectual and psychiatric disabilities, and two patients were diagnosed with only a transient psychiatric impairment during treatment interruption. Meanwhile, 12 patients in the pre-NBS group were diagnosed with neuropsychiatric diseases (six patients with only intellectual disability, five with intellectual and psychiatric disabilities, and one with only psychiatric disability).

Table 3. Comparison of clinical and social parameters.

	NBS Group (n = 68)					Pre-NBS Group (n = 17)		
	20–24 y (n = 22)	25–29 y (n = 19)	30–34 y (n = 14)	35–38 y (n = 13)	Total (%)	39–44 (n = 10) *	45–50 y (n = 7)	Total (%)
Psychiatric status								
normal	20	19	13	12	64 (94%)	7	4	11 (65%)
transient impairment during treatment interruption	2	0	1	0	3 (4%)	0	0	0 (0%)
psychiatric disability	0	0	0	1	1 (1%)	3	3	6 (35%)
Physical characteristics								
normal	19	13	14	11	57 (84%)	5	7	12 (71%)
short stature	1	0	0	0	1 (1%)	1	0	1 (6%)
obesity	2	3	0	1	6 (9%)	2	0	2 (12%)
obesity and short stature	0	2	0	0	2 (3%)	0	0	0 (0%)
leanness	0	1	0	1	2 (3%)	1	0	1 (6%)
unknown	0	0	0	0	0 (0%)	1	0	1 (6%)
Education status								
university	9	10	3	4	26 (38%)	1	1	2 (12%)
technical school	3	5	3	0	11 (16%)	1	0	1 (6%)
high school #	10	2	4	2	18 (26%)	2	2	4 (24%)
junior high school	0	0	0	1	1 (1%)	0	0	0 (0%)
school for individuals with a disability	0	0	0	1	1 (1%)	3	2	5 (30%)
unknown	0	2	4	5	11 (16%)	3	2	5 (30%)
Employment status								
attending school	4	1	0	0	5 (7%)	0	0	0 (0%)
employed	18	17	14	12	61 (90%)	3	4	7 (41%)
unemployed	0	1	0	1	2 (3%)	4	1	5 (30%)
living in a house for individuals with a disability	0	0	0	0	0 (0%)	3	2	5 (30%)
unknown	0	0	0	0	0 (0%)	0	0	0 (0%)
Marital status								
married	0	4	9	6	19 (28%)	2	0	2 (12%)
unmarried or divorce	14	8	4	5	31 (46%)	8	5	13 (76%)
unknown	8	7	1	2	18 (26%)	0	2	2 (12%)

Short stature was defined as a height <160 cm for males and <148 cm for females. Obesity and leanness were defined as BMI >25 and <18.5, respectively. *, A 37-year-old female is included in the group of "39–44 years old" because she did not undergo NBS. #, Graduation from "high school" includes five patients who are still in college.

The relationship between neuropsychiatric symptoms and treatment interruption is described below. In the NBS group, 5 of 21 patients with treatment interruption had a neuropsychiatric disease, while 5 of 47 patients who were continuing treatment had a neuropsychiatric disease. A 35-year-old female patient who had the earliest and longest treatment discontinuation period (for approximately 23 years beginning at an age of 11 years) in the NBS group presented with a psychiatric disability and "moderate-severe intellectual disability" that was the worst intellectual level in the NBS group. Although 5 of 10 patients in the NBS group with a neuropsychiatric disability had a history of treatment discontinuation, the details, such as how long and when treatment discontinued, and Phe levels, were not accurately obtained. On the other hand, in the pre-NBS group, four of five patients with treatment interruption had a neuropsychiatric disease, while 8 of 12 patients who were continuing treatment had a neuropsychiatric disease. From another perspective, 4 of 12 patients with a neuropsychiatric disability had a history of treatment discontinuation. A 42-year-old female in the pre-NBS group who discontinued treatment at 3 years old based on the recommendation of an attending physician, as mentioned above, was unable to be employed, despite her normal intelligence, due to a psychiatric disability induced by intermittent treatment discontinuation for a few decades.

The rate of normal physical size in the NBS group was higher than that in the pre-NBS group, but no obvious differences in physical measurements, including short stature, obesity, or leanness, were observed between the two groups.

Information on education status was obtained for 57 of the 68 patients in the NBS group and 12 of the 17 patients in the pre-NBS group. Fifty-five of 57 (96%) patients in the NBS group had an education level of high school or higher, while 7/12 (58%) patients in the pre-NBS group graduated from high school or higher educational institutions.

Regarding employment status, all but two patients (97%) in the NBS group were employed or attended universities. One of the two unemployed patients was a married female with normal intelligence and was managed to prevent maternal PKU. She was likely a full-time housewife, although this information was not provided. Meanwhile, seven patients (41%) in the pre-NBS group were employed. Five patients each in the pre-NBS group were unemployed or were living in a facility for individuals with a disability. Four of five unemployed patients had intellectual and/or psychiatric disabilities. The other unemployed patient had normal intelligence but also had a tracheostomy due to other respiratory diseases. In summary, all but one of the patients in the NBS group was able to live an independent life, while over half of the patients in the pre-NBS group were not employed or lived in facilities for individuals with disabilities.

Regarding the marital status, 19 of 50 patients in the NBS group were married, while 2 of 15 patients in the pre-NBS group were married.

When given the opportunity to freely describe the patient, many attending physicians stated the difficulty in continuing a Phe-restricted diet, the necessity for lifelong treatment, the need to support medical expenses, and/or the necessity for consultation with internal medicine and psychiatric specialists.

4. Discussion

Our study examined the physical, neurological and social status of adult patients who were diagnosed with PKU before and after NBS in Japan and revealed that NBS obviously contributed to the improvement of long-term outcomes; our results were similar to those of previous reports [1,15–17]. While almost all patients in the NBS group exhibited normal mental development and were able to live an independent life, over half of the patients in the pre-NBS group had neurological and psychiatric problems and were more severely disabled. However, even in the NBS group, 10 patients had intellectual and/or psychiatric disabilities. Because five of them had histories of treatment interruption, continuous and lifelong treatment is essential for good neurological outcomes.

Meanwhile, five patients in the NBS group whose disease remained well-controlled from birth presented with intellectual and/or psychiatric disabilities despite having no history of treatment interruption. In particular, the neurological outcomes of patients in their late 30s (born from 1977 to 1981) were not as good as those in the younger age group. Four of five patients with neuropsychiatric diseases despite continuing the treatment were in their late 30s. This difference is due to less strict target levels of Phe at the beginning stage of NBS [3,18]. In fact, the target levels of plasma Phe concentration were 4–8 mg/dL in babyhood and 4–12 mg/dL in childhood in Japanese guidelines at that time. In addition, because the recommended Phe levels after the age of 6 years were not indicated until the early 1990s, some Japanese physicians considered that dietary therapy could be relaxed and the dietary restriction could be discontinued after patients reached school age. Because the restriction of Phe was not sufficient even before 20 years, a patient aged in the early 20s had a borderline intellectual disability, despite having no history of poor Phe management. As well as this patient, patients who were detected by NBS, even those with proper management, showed poor neurological outcomes in previous studies [16,19]. Hence, in the present guidelines, the restriction of Phe has become stricter.

Namely, not only continuous but also more restricted diet therapy is necessary for good neurological outcomes.

Normal intelligence was observed in some patients in the pre-NBS group despite treatment after onset for unexplained reasons. Additionally, some untreated individuals with classic PKU have normal intelligence despite the elevated plasma Phe concentration [1]. However, the reasons are still unknown. In our study, the symptoms at the onset, what triggered their diagnosis, and when and what type of treatment they had received were not recorded, while our results revealed that their clinical forms were all classic, their age ranged from 39 to 46 years, and one patient had a treatment interruption for 7 years, indicating that the factors constituting a good neurological prognosis are unknown.

Our study also revealed the reasons why patients with PKU discontinued and restarted treatment. Although the unpleasant taste of the special formula is well known [20], treatment interruption was more frequently caused by economic problems in our study. In fact, because the medical public support system for adult patients with PKU has improved since 2015 in Japan, some patients were able to restart treatment. Therefore, lifelong administrative-economic support is necessary to continue treatment. Furthermore, treatment was often neglected due to the self-judgment of being free of symptoms and personal circumstances, such as busy school life and working during adulthood or after childhood. Although many patients detected by Japanese NBS are strictly controlled in childhood by physicians, nutritionists, medical staff, and family, they are released from strict management after adulthood due to independence from those supporters. Therefore, adult patients tend to neglect regular visits and strict dietary therapy due to poor subjective symptoms, and neurological symptoms progress over a chronic course. On the other hand, the primary reason for restarting treatment was pregnancy and the prevention of maternal PKU. Therefore, we strongly suggest that appropriate and continuous patient education is the most effective method to prevent loss to follow-up.

In our study, psychiatric disabilities were likely to progress in the later period of life. One of the reasons may be a difference in the quality of disease management between childhood and adulthood, as mentioned above. In fact, some patients present with psychiatric disabilities after adulthood due to inadequate self-management or treatment intermittence despite having normal intelligence and receiving higher education in childhood. Additionally, it was previously reported that neuropsychiatric symptoms are more prevalent in older adults with PKU [21]. Namely, PKU is considered a progressive disease even after adulthood. Higher blood levels of Phe inhibit myelination in early childhood and functionally impair myelin in late childhood or adulthood, even after normal myelination [22]. Thus, continuous treatment is important for favorable neuropsychiatric outcomes.

Regarding physical development, no obvious differences were detected between the NBS and pre-NBS groups. Nevertheless, optimal growth outcomes were not attained in a previous study, even with advances in dietary treatments [23]. Although our study did not indicate major issues related to growth, physical development should be continuously evaluated for each individual with PKU.

Our results also indicated that the transition to an adult internal medicine department is not easy at this time in Japan. In fact, this issue has been observed in not only Japan but also other countries [24] and for not only PKU patients but also patients with other rare diseases [25]. The explanation for this finding is that internal medicine physicians for adults have little knowledge of PKU or are unable to appropriately treat this disease. In addition and very importantly, patients with PKU realize this limitation and generally prefer to be treated by pediatricians who are experts in PKU care and treatment. Furthermore, patients feel comfortable visiting a place where they know the care providers rather than a new and strange facility. Therefore, the transition to adult department is a major issue for all adult patients with PKU. Furthermore, the issue of the transition and when to make transition have not been described yet in Japanese guidelines, although preparations for the transition from pediatrics to adult internal medicine should begin at approximately 12 years of age based on European guidelines [18,26]. Namely, transitions are likely to be delayed in Japan compared with Europe.

Finally, our study may have some limitations. Only patients who were treated with Phe-free formula and could be traced after adulthood were recruited for our study. According to the annual report of Japanese NBS, approximately 400 adult patients were estimated to be diagnosed with PKU during the period from 1977 to 1996. However, in the present study, only 68 patients were enrolled in the NBS group. Our study did not include a considerable number of adult patients with PKU who no longer received treatment at the hospital, discontinued treatment with Phe-free formula, were treated with only BH_4, and died before adulthood. Furthermore, because the participants in this study had continuously or intermittently ordered the special formula, they were willing to be treated even after reaching adulthood. Therefore, our results might be shifted to better outcomes of PKU than the actual situation. Nevertheless, our results are useful for many Asian physicians because the long-term outcomes of East Asian patients with PKU have not been well understood to date. Improvements in the patient registration, follow-up and medical support systems for adult and pediatric patients with PKU will be essential for achieving lifelong favorable outcomes.

5. Conclusions

The long-term outcomes of adult patients with PKU detected by NBS were much more favorable than those of patients in the pre-NBS group in Japan, as previously reported in other countries. However, some patients, even those who underwent early detection using NBS, with histories of treatment intermittence suffered from neuropsychiatric symptoms. Lifelong and strict management is essential to maintain a good prognosis for patients with PKU.

Author Contributions: Conceptualization, K.Y. (Kenji Yamada), K.A. and S.Y.; Methodology, K.Y. (Kenji Yamada) and S.Y.; Software, K.Y. (Kenji Yamada) and K.Y. (Kazunori Yokoyama); Validation, K.Y. (Kenji Yamada) and K.Y. (Kazunori Yokoyama); Formal Analysis, K.Y. (Kenji Yamada) and K.Y. (Kazunori Yokoyama); Investigation, K.Y. (Kenji Yamada) and S.Y.; Data Cu-ration, K.Y. (Kenji Yamada) and K.Y. (Kazunori Yokoyama); Writing–Original Draft Preparation, K.Y. (Kenji Yamada); Writing–Review and Editing, K.Y. (Kazunori Yokoyama), K.A., T.T. and S.Y.; Visualization, K.Y. (Kenji Yamada); Supervision, K.A., T.T. and S.Y.; Project Administration, K.A., T.T. and S.Y.; Funding Acquisition, K.Y. (Kenji Yamada) and S.Y. All authors have read and agreed to the published version of the manuscript.

Funding: This report was partially supported by AMED (grant numbers JP16ek0109050, JP19ek0109276, and JP20ek0109482) and JSPS KAKENHI (grant numbers 19K08300 and 19K08347). The authors confirm that the sponsors had no role in the study; the content of the article was not influenced by the sponsors.

Institutional Review Board Statement: The study was conducted according to the guidelines of the Declaration of Helsinki, and approved by the Institutional Review Board of Shimane University on 13 October 2016 (protocol code #20160915-2 and date of approval).

Informed Consent Statement: Patient consent was waived because this study is retrospective based on already-existing data using questionnaire for attending doctor and because it is difficult to obtain informed consent of some patients due to not visiting the hospital within the research period. However, this study concept and implementation are widely announced on our university website

Acknowledgments: We thank Y. Okano (Okano Kodomo Clinic, Izumi), T. Takahashi (Takahashi Clinic, Kobe), M. Takahashi (Isesaki Municipal Hospital, Isesaki), T. Fukao (Gifu University, Gifu), Y. Watanabe (Kurume University, Kurume), M. Araki (Kochi University, Kochi), M. Furujo (Okayama Medical Center, Okayama), J. Toyama (Nishiniigata Chuo Hospital, Niigata), H. Motizuki (Saitama Children's Medical Center, Saitama), C. Numakura (Yamagata University, Yamagata), K. Kosugiyama (Teine Keijinkai Hospital, Sapporo), A. Noguchi (Akita University, Akita), H. Awano and M. Yagi (Kobe University, Kobe), K. Shiota (St. Luke's International Hospital, Tokyo), A. Matsunaga and T. Fushimi (Chiba Children's Hospital, Chiba), K. Hamaguchi (Kuramochi Hospital, Tochigi), T. Yorifuji,

(Osaka City General Hospital, Osaka), D. Tokuhara, H. Shintaku, K. Hamasaki, and M. Saito (Osaka City University, Osaka), M. Oshio (Kyushu Hospital, Kitakyushu), Y. Hasegawa (Tokyo Metropolitan Children's Medical Center, Tokyo), O. Sakamoto (Tohoku University, Sendai), T. Ito and Y. Nakajima (Fujita Health University, Toyoake), T. Asano (Nippon Medical School Chibahokusoh Hospital, Inzai), M. Ishige and E. Ogawa (Tokyo Health Service Association, Tokyo), K. Yoshimura and R. Tsurusawa (Fukuoka University, Fukuoka), M. Owada (Tokyo Health Service Association, Tokyo), M. Shiroo (Kyusyu Hospital Kitakyusyu), M. Inoue (Misakae No Sono, Isohaya), and T. Kakiba (Matsue Red Cross Hospital, Matsue) for participating in and assisting with our study.

Conflicts of Interest: The authors declare no conflict of interest.

Abbreviations

NBS	newborn screening
PKU	phenylketonuria
PAH	phenylalanine hydroxylase
Phe	phenylalanine
BH_4	tetrahydrobiopterin
HPA	hyperphenylalaninemia;
IQ	intelligence quotient

References

1. Mitchell, J.J.; Trakadis, Y.J.; Scriver, C.R. Phenylalanine hydroxylase deficiency. *Genet. Med.* **2011**, *13*, 697–707. [CrossRef]
2. Ozalp, I.; Coşkun, T.; Tokatli, A.; Kalkanoğlu, H.S.; Dursun, A.; Tokol, S.; Köksal, G.; Ozgüc, M.; Köse, R. Newborn PKU screening in Turkey: At present and organization for future. *Turk. J. Pediatr.* **2001**, *43*, 97–101. [PubMed]
3. Vockley, J.; Andersson, H.C.; Antshel, K.M.; Braverman, N.E.; Burton, B.K.; Frazier, D.M.; Mitchell, J.; Smith, W.E.; Thompson, B.H.; Berry, S.A. Phenylalanine hydroxylase deficiency: Diagnosis and management guideline. *Genet. Med.* **2014**, *16*, 188–200. [PubMed]
4. Shibata, N.; Hasegawa, Y.; Yamada, K.; Kobayashi, H.; Purevsuren, J.; Yang, Y.; Dung, V.C.; Khanh, N.N.; Verma, I.C.; Bijarnia-Mahay, S.; et al. Diversity in the incidence and spectrum of organic acidemias, fatty acid oxidation disorders, and amino acid disorders in Asian countries: Selective screening vs. expanded newborn screening. *Mol. Genet. Metab. Rep.* **2018**, *16*, 5–10. [CrossRef] [PubMed]
5. Aoki, K. Long term follow-up of patients with inborn errors of metabolism detected by the newborn screening program in Japan. *Southeast Asian J. Trop. Med. Public Health* **2003**, *34* (Suppl. S3), 19–23. [PubMed]
6. Lord, J.; Thomason, M.J.; Littlejohns, P.; Chalmers, R.A.; Bain, M.D.; Addison, G.M.; Wilcox, A.H.; Seymour, C.A. Secondary analysis of economic data: A review of cost-benefit studies of neonatal screening for phenylketonuria. *J. Epidemiol. Community Health* **1999**, *53*, 179–186. [CrossRef] [PubMed]
7. Dhondt, J.L.; Farriaux, J.P.; Sailly, J.C.; Lebrun, T. Economic evaluation of cost-benefit ratio of neonatal screening procedure for phenylketonuria and hypothyroidism. *J. Inherit. Metab. Dis.* **1991**, *14*, 633–639. [CrossRef]
8. Koch, R.; Burton, B.; Hoganson, G.; Peterson, R.; Rhead, W.; Rouse, B.; Scott, R.; Wolff, J.; Stern, A.M.; Guttler, F.; et al. Phenylketonuria in adulthood: A collaborative study. *J. Inherit. Metab. Dis.* **2002**, *25*, 333–346. [CrossRef] [PubMed]
9. Moyle, J.J.; Fox, A.M.; Arthur, M.; Bynevelt, M.; Burnett, J.R. Meta-analysis of neuropsychological symptoms of adolescents and adults with PKU. *Neuropsychol. Rev.* **2007**, *17*, 91–101. [CrossRef]
10. Waisbren, S.E.; Noel, K.; Fahrbach, K.; Cella, C.; Frame, D.; Dorenbaum, A.; Levy, H. Phenylalanine blood levels and clinical outcomes in phenylketonuria: A systematic literature review and meta-analysis. *Mol. Genet. Metab.* **2007**, *92*, 63–70. [CrossRef]
11. Burton, B.K.; Leviton, L.; Vespa, H.; Coon, H.; Longo, N.; Lundy, B.D.; Johnson, M.; Angelino, A.; Hamosh, A.; Bilder, D. A diversified approach for PKU treatment: Routine screening yields high incidence of psychiatric distress in phenylketonuria clinics. *Mol. Genet. Metab.* **2013**, *108*, 8–12. [CrossRef]
12. Antshel, K.M. ADHD, learning, and academic performance in phenylketonuria. *Mol. Genet. Metab.* **2010**, *99* (Suppl. S1), S52–S58. [CrossRef] [PubMed]
13. Aoki, K.; Ohwada, M.; Kitagawa, T. Long-term follow-up study of patients with phenylketonuria detected by the newborn screening programme in Japan. *J. Inherit. Metab. Dis.* **2007**, *30*, 608. [CrossRef] [PubMed]
14. Aoki, K.; Wada, Y. Outcome of the patients detected by newborn screening in Japan. *Acta Paediatr. Jpn.* **1988**, *30*, 429–434. [CrossRef] [PubMed]
15. Trefz, F.; Maillot, F.; Motzfeldt, K.; Schwarz, M. Adult phenylketonuria outcome and management. *Mol. Genet. Metab.* **2011**, *104*, S26–S30. [CrossRef] [PubMed]
16. Burlina, A.P.; Lachmann, R.H.; Manara, R.; Cazzorla, C.; Celato, A.; van Spronsen, F.J.; Burlina, A. The neurological and psychological phenotype of adult patients with early-treated phenylketonuria: A systematic review. *J. Inherit. Metab. Dis.* **2019**, *42*, 209–219. [CrossRef] [PubMed]

17. Nardecchia, F.; Manti, F.; Chiarotti, F.; Carducci, C.; Carducci, C.; Leuzzi, V. Neurocognitive and neuroimaging outcome of early treated young adult PKU patients: A longitudinal study. *Mol. Genet. Metab.* **2015**, *115*, 84–90. [CrossRef]
18. Van Wegberg, A.M.J.; MacDonald, A.; Ahring, K.; Bélanger-Quintana, A.; Blau, N.; Bosch, A.M.; Burlina, A.; Campistol, J.; Feillet, F.; Giżewska, M.; et al. The complete European guidelines on phenylketonuria: Diagnosis and treatment. *Orphanet J. Rare Dis.* **2017**, *12*, 162. [CrossRef]
19. Hofman, D.L.; Champ, C.L.; Lawton, C.L.; Henderson, M.; Dye, L. A systematic review of cognitive functioning in early treated adults with phenylketonuria. *Orphanet J. Rare Dis.* **2018**, *13*, 150. [CrossRef]
20. Owada, M.; Aoki, K.; Kitagawa, T. Taste preferences and feeding behaviour in children with phenylketonuria on a semisynthetic diet. *Eur. J. Pediatr.* **2000**, *159*, 846–850. [CrossRef]
21. Bilder, D.A.; Kobori, J.A.; Cohen-Pfeffer, J.L.; Johnson, E.M.; Jurecki, E.R.; Grant, M.L. Neuropsychiatric comorbidities in adults with phenylketonuria: A retrospective cohort study. *Mol. Genet. Metab.* **2017**, *121*, 1–8. [CrossRef] [PubMed]
22. Anderson, P.J.; Leuzzi, V. White matter pathology in phenylketonuria. *Mol. Genet. Metab.* **2010**, *99* (Suppl. S1), S3–S9. [CrossRef] [PubMed]
23. Ilgaz, F.; Pinto, A.; Gökmen-Özel, H.; Rocha, J.C.; van Dam, E.; Ahring, K.; Bélanger-Quintana, A.; Dokoupil, K.; Karabulut, E.; MacDonald, A. Long-Term Growth in Phenylketonuria: A Systematic Review and Meta-Analysis. *Nutrients* **2019**, *11*, 2070. [CrossRef]
24. Demirkol, M.; Giżewska, M.; Giovannini, M.; Walter, J. Follow up of phenylketonuria patients. *Mol. Genet. Metab.* **2011**, *104*, S31–S39. [CrossRef] [PubMed]
25. Mazzucato, M.; Visonà Dalla Pozza, L.; Minichiello, C.; Manea, S.; Barbieri, S.; Toto, E.; Vianello, A.; Facchin, P. The Epidemiology of Transition into Adulthood of Rare Diseases Patients: Results from a Population-Based Registry. *Int. J. Environ. Res. Public Health* **2018**, *15*, 2212. [CrossRef] [PubMed]
26. Mütze, U.; Roth, A.; Weigel, J.F.; Beblo, S.; Baerwald, C.G.; Bührdel, P.; Kiess, W. Transition of young adults with phenylketonuria from pediatric to adult care. *J. Inherit. Metab. Dis.* **2011**, *34*, 701–709. [CrossRef]

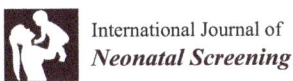

Article

Clinical and Genetic Characteristics of Patients with Mild Hyperphenylalaninemia Identified by Newborn Screening Program in Japan

Shino Odagiri [1], Daijiro Kabata [2], Shogo Tomita [2], Satoshi Kudo [1], Tomoko Sakaguchi [1], Noriko Nakano [1], Kouji Yamamoto [3], Haruo Shintaku [4] and Takashi Hamazaki [1,*]

1. Department of Pediatrics, Osaka City University Graduate School of Medicine, Osaka 545-8585, Japan; shino.taniguchi@gmail.com (S.O.); kudo-satoshi@jfe-eng.co.jp (S.K.); saka-tomo@med.osaka-cu.ac.jp (T.S.); nakano.noriko@med.osaka-cu.ac.jp (N.N.)
2. Department of Medical Statistics, Osaka City University Graduate School of Medicine, Osaka 545-8585, Japan; kabata.daijiro@med.osaka-cu.ac.jp (D.K.); ssfrfc3k@icloud.com (S.T.)
3. Department of Biostatistics, Yokohama City University School of Medicine, Yokohama 236-0004, Japan; kouji_y@yokohama-cu.ac.jp
4. Donated Course "Disability Medicine and Regenerative Medicine", Osaka City University Graduate School of Medicine, Osaka 545-8585, Japan; shintakuh@med.osaka-cu.ac.jp
* Correspondence: hammer@med.osaka-cu.ac.jp; Tel.: +81-6-6645-3815

Abstract: Phenylketonuria (PKU) and hyperphenylalaninemia (HPA), both identified in newborn screening, are attributable to variants in *PAH*. Reportedly, the p.R53H(c.158G>A) variant is common in patients with HPA in East Asia. Here, we aimed to define the association between p.R53H and HPA phenotype, and study the long-term outcome of patients with HPA carrying p.R53H. We retrospectively reviewed the genotype in 370 patients detected by newborn screening, and identified the phenotype in 280 (117, HPA; 163, PKU). p.R413P(c.1238G>C) was the most frequently found ($n = 117$, 31.6%) variant, followed by *p.R53H* ($n = 89$, 24.1%). The odds ratio for heterozygous p.R53H to cause HPA was 48.3 (95% CI 19.410–120.004). Furthermore, we assessed the non-linear association between the phenylalanine (Phe) value and elapsed time using the follow-up data of the blood Phe levels of 73 patients with HPA carrying p.R53H. The predicted levels peaked at 161.9 µmol (95% CI 152.088–172.343) at 50–60 months of age and did not exceed 360 µmol/L during the 210-month long observation period. The findings suggest that patients with HPA, carrying p.R53H, do not need frequent Phe monitoring as against those with PKU. Our study provides convincing evidence to determine clinical management of patients detected through newborn screening in Japan.

Keywords: phenylketonuria; hyperphenylalaninemia; phenylalanine hydroxylase; genetic analysis; neonatal screening; genotype–phenotype correlation

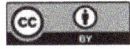

1. Introduction

Phenylketonuria (PKU) and hyperphenylalaninemia (HPA) are autosomal recessive disorders characterized by the deficiency of hepatic phenylalanine hydroxylase (PAH) [1]. This enzyme is encoded by *PAH* located on chromosome 12q, and comprising 13 exons and 12 introns. The genotype–phenotype correlations in PKU have been demonstrated using predicted PAH activity, which is the average in vitro residual PAH activity of two alleles [2].

The severity of the disorder is diverse, ranging from HPA to classical PKU that is characterized by high blood phenylalanine (Phe) levels [3]. The European and US guidelines for PKU recommend studying its molecular genetics and accumulating the data about correlations between the genotype and clinical phenotype [4,5]. Furthermore, more than 1100 variants of *PAH* have been recorded in the locus-specific database PAHvdb (http://www.biopku.org/pah/, accessed on 1 March 2021). However, these data are mainly gathered from European patients. The frequency of *PAH* variants in Japanese and other East Asian populations is different from that in Europeans. Therefore, recording data on the genotype–phenotype correlation in Japanese patients with PKU is required.

In Japan, a nationwide newborn screening (NBS) for PKU was launched in 1977. The current screening cut-off level for Phe on dried blood spots is set >120 μmol/L. When patients with PKU and related disorders are identified via NBS, their clinical phenotypes are classified as follows: (1) tetrahydrobiopterin (BH4) deficiency is ruled out by pteridine analysis and measurement of dihydropteridine reductase activity, (2) PAH deficiency is classified by pretreatment-Phe levels, and (3) Patients with <60 μmol/L Phe level are diagnosed with HPA while those with >360 μmol/L are further classified as BH4-responsive mild PKU or classical PKU based on BH4 loading test.

According to the integrative Japanese Genome Variation Database (iJGVD, https://ijgvd.megabank.tohoku.ac.jp, accessed on 18 February 2021), the allele frequency of p.R53H in the general Japanese population was reported to be as high as 5% [6]. Several studies have reported that p.R53H is associated with HPA phenotype [3,4,7–9]. On the contrary, a few reports exist that correlates PKU with p.R53H [9,10].

In this study, we retrospectively reviewed the genotype–phenotype correlation of 370 patients who were diagnosed with PKU or HPA through NBS in Japan. Consequently, we found that the p.R53H genotype was associated with HPA phenotype, but not with that of PKU. Further, 73 of the patients with HPA carrying the p.R53H variant displayed stable blood Phe levels without needs of permanent treatments during the long-term follow-up. Our findings are especially useful for determining clinical management of such patients in Japan and other East Asian countries.

2. Materials and Methods

2.1. Study Design and Participants

This study was approved by the Institutional Review Board of Osaka City University Graduate School of Medicine (Osaka, Japan) (#3687). Written informed consent for the genetic analyses was obtained from all patients or their parents/guardians. The study included 370 Japanese patients analyzed for *PAH* at our facility during January 1998–March 2017, and for secondary examinations of HPA by NBS. We retrospectively reviewed the medical records of the patients to analyze their phenotype and genotype characteristics. The criterion for PKU phenotype was blood Phe level >600 μmol/L, and that for HPA phenotype was 120–600 μmol/L without Phe-restriction diet. Furthermore, we analyzed the genotype–phenotype correlation with *p.R53H* and the follow-up data of blood Phe levels of patients with HPA carrying *p.R53H* from the retrieved medical records.

2.2. Statistical Analysis

To evaluate whether the p.R53H variant is the cause underlying the HPA phenotype, we performed multivariate logistic regression analysis in the PKU (including HPA) pediatric patients who underwent genetic analysis using the variable indicating presence or absence of the HPA phenotype as the outcome and the number of the p.R53H variants as the explanatory variable. This regression model was adjusted the following covariates; the presence of the p.R413P, p.R241C(c.721C>T), p.R111*(c.721C>T), IVS4-1G>A(c.442-1G>A), p.R243Q(c.728G>A), p.T278I(c.833C>T), p.R252W(c.754C>T), p.Ex6-96A>G(c.611A>G) and variants in the *PAH* gene and sex. The multiple imputation was conducted to impute the missing values for all variables.

Furthermore, in order to assess the change of Phe level over time, we performed non-linear regression analysis with the Huber–White robust sandwich estimator of variance–covariance matrix. The robust estimator considers dependence in repeated measures within a single patient. Additionally, non-linear restricted-cubic-spline was conducted to assess the non-linear association between Phe level and the elapsed time. In this mode, Phe levels were used with natural-log transformation to satisfy the assumption of normality of the error distribution.

All statistical tests were performed two-sided with 5% significance level. The analyses were conducted using R (https://www.r-project.org/foundation/, accessed on 21 December 2020) (https://cran.r-project.org/, accessed on 21 December 2020).

3. Results

We retrospectively examined the genotype and clinical phenotypic characteristics of the 370 subjects with PAH deficiency and blood Phe levels of >120 μmol/L detected through NBS. Frequency of variants in *PAH* observed are summarized in Figure 1, and all PAH variations (*n* = 370) found in the study cohort are shown in Table S1. Briefly, p.R413P was most frequently found (*n* = 117, 31.6%), followed by p.R53H (*n* = 89, 24.1%), p.R241C (*n* = 53, 14.3%), p.R111* (*n* = 47, 12.7%), and IVS4-1G>A (*n* = 44, 11.9%). Five patients had large deletions involving exons 5 and 6. In all, no variant was identified in three patients while one variant was identified in 27; two in 238; three in 11; and four in two. Phenotypes were identified in 280/370 patients, wherein HPA was identified in 117 and PKU in 163.

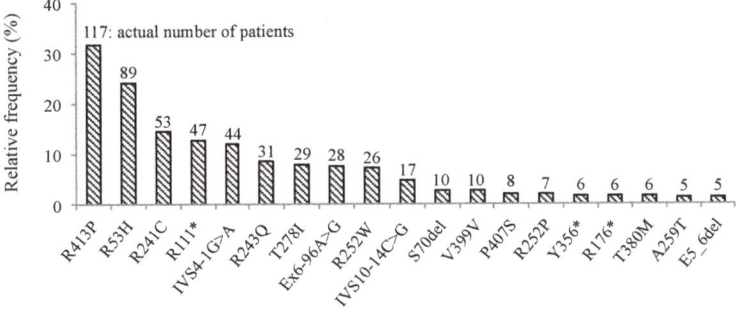

Figure 1. Frequency of *PAH* variants in 370 patients with elevated Phe levels detected by mass screening. Percentage of patients with mutations in *PAH* was detected by direct sequencing or multiplex ligation-dependent probe amplification (MLPA) in all the participants enrolled in this study. Numbers at the top of the vertical bars represent the actual number of patients with each mutation. Infrequent mutations have been omitted. Phe; phenylalanine, *PAH*; gene encoding phenylalanine hydroxylase, * stop codon.

We, next, compared the frequency of the p.R53H variant between patients with HPA and PKU (Figure 2A). Consequently, we found that the frequency of p.R53H in those with HPA phenotype was 61.0% (74/117). From these, three were homozygous for p.R53H while 71 were heterozygous. The frequency of p.R53H in the patients with PKU phenotype was 6.7% (11/163). Of them, one was homozygous for p.R53H while 10 were heterozygous. In order to validate that the p.R53H variant is associated with HPA phenotype rather than that of PKU, we performed multivariate logistic regression analysis. Accordingly, we adjusted the influence of the other alleles frequently found in this population. The odds ratio for patients with heterozygous p.R53H to develop HPA phenotype was 48.3 (95% confidence interval [CI] 19.410–120.004) (Figure 2B). The odds ratio for patients with homozygous p.R53H to develop HPA phenotype was 26.2 (95% CI 2.054–334.832). This result demonstrated that patients with homozygous or heterozygous p.R53H variant are more likely to manifest HPA rather than PKU.

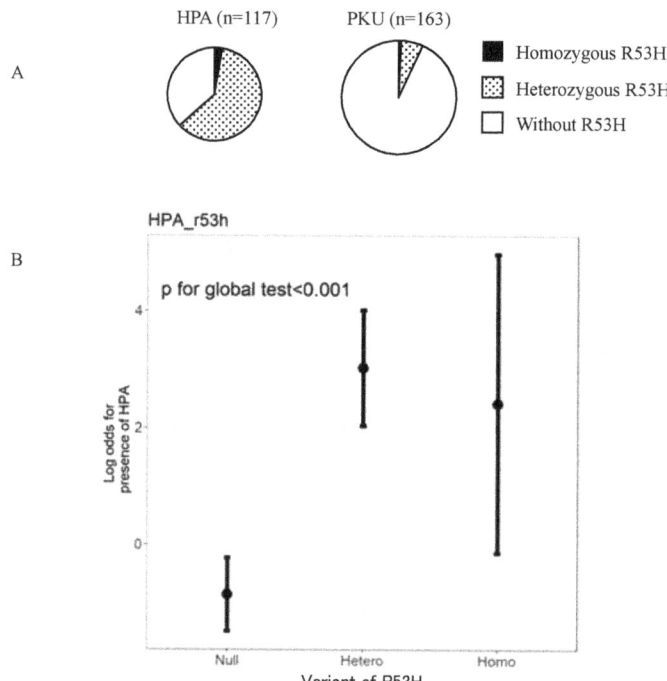

Figure 2. p.R53H variant is observed at a higher frequency in patients with HPA phenotype than in patients with PKU phenotype. (**A**) Number of patients with R53H variant in PAH (p.R53H) in each of the 280 patients with a known phenotype of either HPA or PKU. (**B**) Odds ratios for patients with no, heterozygous, and homozygous p.R53H variant to develop HPA phenotype. HPA, hyperphenylalaninemia; PKU, Phenylketonuria.

We further examined the status of p.R53H in the 11 patients with PKU. Consequently, we found that one patient had four variants, homozygous p.R53H and homozygous p.R158W; seven patients had three variants, heterozygous p.R53H and two other variants, p.R413P/p.R252W, p.R111*/p.R252W, p.R111*/IVS9+1G>A(c.969+1G>A), IVS4-1G>A/p.R252W, p.R252W/p.EX6-96A>G, p.R252W/p.V399V(c.1197A>T), and p.P407S (c.1219C>T)/p.R158W(c.472C>T). Therefore, the presence of these variants other than p.R53H explains the manifestation of PKU in eight of the 11 identified patients [11–18]. The remaining three had only one heterozygous variant (p.R413P, p.R111*, and p.R252W) other than p.R53H.

To determine which of the genetic variants were responsible for HPA phenotype, we analyzed them in the 117 patients with HPA. We categorized the patients into three groups based on their phenotypes predicted from the previously reported genotype–phenotype correlations (Table 1). The left column lists 74 patients with HPA who carried the p.R53H variant. In these patients, genetic variants that are known to cause PKU, such as p.R413P and p.R243Q, were recurrently found. On the contrary, only three of 74 patients had the p.R241C variant, which was associated with BH4-responsive PKU. Patients homozygous for p.R53H were not found in our study. The middle column shows cases carrying variants associated with HPA except for p.R53H. The right column shows remaining cases carrying variants with predicted PKU or unknown phenotype. In this group, p.R241C variant was found in 18 patients. Three patients with homozygous p.R241C manifested the HPA phenotype, while only one patient with same the genotype manifested PKU phenotype (data not shown).

Table 1. PAH variants identified in 117 patients with HPA phenotype.

Variants with R53H (n = 74)		Variants without R53H (n = 43)			
		Predicted HPA phenotype		Predicted PKU phenotype or unknown phenotype	
Genotype	n	Genotype	n	Genotype	n
R53H/R413P	15	R71H/T278I	1	R241C/R241C	3
R53H/R243Q	6	A132V/R413P	1	R241C/S70del	2
R53H/T278I	6	A132V/	1	R241C/P407S	1
R53H/Ex6-96A>G	5	R297C/ IVS4-1G>A	1	R241C/ IVS4-1G>A	1
R53H/IVS4-1G>A	4	A373T/R241C	1	R241C/Ex6-96A>G	1
R53H/R252W	4	A373T/T380M	1	R241C/R243Q	1
R53H/E5_6del	3	A373T/R413P	1	R241C/R252P	1
R53H/E3del4bp	3	Q375E/delS70	1	R241C/T278I	3
R53H/R111*	3	Q375E/ IVS4-1G>A	1	R241C/R413P	2
R53H/R241C	3	V379A/R111*	1	R241C/P281A	1
R53H/E6del	2	V379A/R252W	1	R241C/	2
R53H/V399V	2	T380M/IVS10-14C>G	3	R413P/	2
R53H/A259T	1	T380M/R111*	1	F55L/Y154D	1
R53H/S70del	1	T380M/ IVS4-1G>A	1	R243Q/	1
R53H/F402I	1	F402I/R252W	1	K431N/	1
R53H/IVS10-14C>G	1	A403V/S16*	1	S67C/	1
R53H/IVS10-1C>G	1	D415N/R353W	1		
R53H/L421T	1				
R53H/P281L	1				
R53H/R176X	1				
R53H/R243*	1				
R53H/R408W	1				
R53H/R413C	1				
R53H/V412P	1				
R53H/A132V/R413P	1				
R53H/	5				

There are no studies that report the long-term follow-up data of patients with HPA carrying p.R53H. We, thus, investigated the detailed clinicopathological characteristics of these patients. In the 74 patients with HPA carrying p.R53H, we excluded one patient carrying two pathogenic variants other than p.R53H. We analyzed the blood Phe levels in 73 patients (Figure 3). These patients included 31 males, 40 females, and two patients for whom gender data were not available. The observation period was of 0–210 months (median: 33 months). The mean of their blood Phe levels was 150 ± 30 µmol/L, and the maximum level found was 340 µmol/L. No patients had impaired mental and physical development. Furthermore, using the blood Phe levels at each visit of these patients and 635 data counts, we assessed the non-linear association between the Phe level and the elapsed time. The predicted Phe level at 0 month was 136.470 µmol/L (95% CI 131.491–141.638), but the Phe level peaked at 161.899 µmol/L (95% CI 152.088–172.343) at 50–60 months. Thereafter, the predicted Phe level gradually decreased to 106.246 µmol/L (95% CI 80.829–139.656) at 200 months of age. The predicted Phe levels did not exceed 360 µmol/L throughout the observation period.

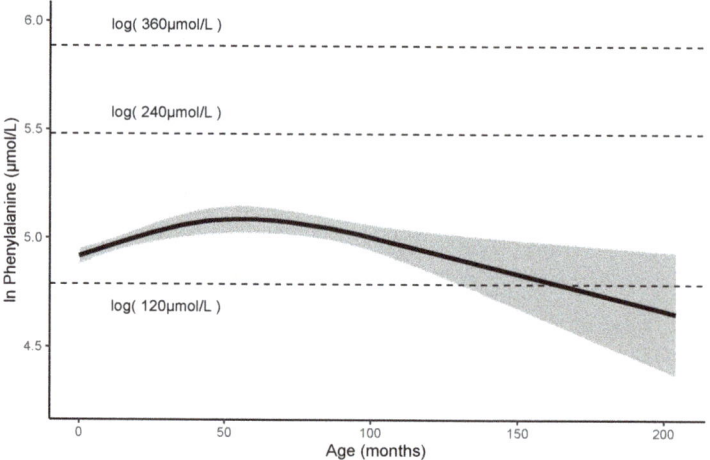

Figure 3. Predicted Phe levels until 200-month-olds are less than 360 μmol/L in patients with HPA carrying p.R53H.

Changes in the predicted Phe levels in the patients. Solid line represents mean value; gray area represents 95% confidence interval. HPA, hyperphenylalaninemia; Phe; phenylalanine.

4. Discussion

We examined the genotypes of 370 patients with HPA or PKU identified by NBS in Japan. Consequently, we found that the p.R53H variant was recurrent in patients with HPA. Our study rigorously demonstrated that carrying compound heterozygous p.R53H and classical PKU-associated variants can predict HPA phenotype. Patients with PKU, carrying p.R53H, were likely to have two other pathogenic variants. Consequently, we found that the levels were maintained lower than 360 μmol/L until adolescence in the absence of Phe-restriction dietary treatment. Our findings provide convincing evidence that can help plan clinical management of patients detected through NBS in Japan.

As shown in Figure 1, the most common variants identified in this study were p.R413P, p.R53H, and p.R241C. A few East Asian countries, namely Japan, China, Taiwan, and Korea, share a common spectrum of *PAH* variants [11,12,17,19,20]. The variants—p.R243Q, p.EX6-96A>G, p.R241C, and p.R413P—have been frequently detected in the these countries. Further, five variants—p.V399V, p.R111*, p.Y356X(c.1068C>A), IVS4-1G>A, and p.T278I—were shared with each other [12,17]. Allele frequency of p.R53H in the general population is 1.6% in the whole of East Asia, and 2.57% and 4.7% in Korea and Japan, respectively [21,22]. In case of patients detected through NBS, the allele frequency of p.R53H is 12.6% (93/740) in our study, and 1.27% and 2.11% in Korea and Taiwan, respectively [12,17]. Our study predicted the average Phe level for screening positive newborns carrying compound heterozygous p.R53H and other pathogenic variants to be 136.470 μmol/L (95% CI 131.491–141.638). In case of Korea and Taiwan, blood Phe levels of 240–599 μmol/L are used to define HPA; possibly, this is the reason why the p.R53H variant is less frequently detected in their affected populations [12,17]. The frequency of variants and genotypes in Japan is different from that recently published by Hillert et al. [23]. We considered that these differences were made because their study was based on information from only 55 patients.

In this study, 6.7% patients with PKU carried p.R53H (allele frequency, approximately 4%) that is close to 4.7% in the Japanese general population, as mentioned above [21]. This fact also suggested that the p.R53H variant is not directly associated with PKU phenotype. In order to explain the pathogenesis of PKU, these 11 patients must have two other pathogenic variants in addition to p.R53H. However, we found that three of them carried only one other pathogenic variant. In these three patients we further performed multiple ligation-dependent probe amplification (MLPA) to exclude the possibility of large deletions. It should be noted that some genetic variants could not be identified even with the available methods. In previous studies, the detection rates of pathogenic variants among biochemically confirmed PKU cases were 96% (318/330) in China, 98% (139/142) in Taiwan, and 86.7% (137/158) in Korea [8,12,13]. Therefore, it is reasonable to assume that one other variant has not yet been identified in those patients who carry only one pathogenic variant other than p.R53H.

In an analysis of 512 people in the Japanese general population, 48 people (allele frequency, 4.7%) were heterozygous for p.R53H [21]. These heterozygotes displayed an average 19% increase in plasma Phe levels compared to wildtype homozygotes. Interestingly, Choi in Korea reported that the father of a patient with HPA was homozygous for p.R53H but did not manifest HPA [22]. Consistent with these reports, in our study, patients homozygous for p.R53H were not detected by NBS. Our study revealed that patients with HPA and the p.R53H variant frequently carried compound heterozygous classical PKU-associated variant, such as p.R413P, p.R243Q, and p.T278I (Table 1). They were less likely to have the compound heterozygous mild PKU-associated variant, such as p.R241C. A study using COS cells has reported the residual enzyme activities of p.R413P, p.R53H, and p.R241C as 1%, 79%, and 49%, respectively [12]. Collectively, it is reasonable to assume that the combination of variants with high residual enzyme activity will not exceed 120 µmol/L Phe levels to be detected through NBS.

With respect to the cut-off value of Phe levels set for NBS, there are contradictory views; some argue that this cut-off value should be set higher because the current value detects people as PKU-affected even though they do not require treatment. However, patients with BH4 deficiency present around 120 µmol/L Phe levels [24]. Therefore, we consider that the current cut-off value should not be changed such that patients with BH4 deficiency who sometimes maintain low Phe levels are not missed during the screening process. Furthermore, DNAJC12 deficiency that manifests HPA phenotype but not *PAH* variant or BH4 deficiency has been reported earlier [25]. Further, patients with DNAJC12 deficiency who were diagnosed early and accordingly treated showed normal development, while permanent neurological damage was observed with delayed diagnosis. Since p.R53H is present at a high frequency in the Japanese general population [21], it is possible that patients with DNAJC12 deficiency carry this variant. When patients with p.R53H have persistently high Phe levels and exhibit neurological symptoms, such as developmental delay and behavioral disorder, DNAJC12 deficiency should be considered for differential diagnosis.

Since there are no guidelines for HPA in Japan, patients with this condition are also monitored according to the guidelines for PKU. The European guidelines for PKU recommend frequent measurements of blood Phe levels; weekly up to the age of 12 months, followed by fortnightly till 12 years, and monthly for >12 years [4]. The current Japanese follow-up guidelines of PKU recommend that patients undergo measurement of blood Phe levels every four weeks until elementary school entrance [26]. We found that the predicted Phe levels in patients with HPA carrying p.R53H never exceeded 360 µmol/L without Phe-restricted diet until 200 month of age (Figure 2). These facts suggest that patients with HPA do not require frequent follow-ups. Further, we recommend that guidelines be developed on a priority basis for patients with HPA. In patients with PKU, first trimester of pregnancy should be monitored since the Phe levels tend to elevate during this period [4]. According to the European and US guidelines, when the untreated blood Phe level of women of childbearing-age with PKU is 120–360 µmol/L, treatment is unnecessary [4,5]. Extrapolating our study findings, we expect the blood Phe levels of pregnant women with HPA carrying p.R53H to not exceed 360 µmol/L during pregnancy. Further, our findings suggest that Phe-restricted diet and frequent follow-ups are not necessary for such patients even during pregnancy.

There are several limitations associated with the present study. Owing to its retrospective nature, the protocol for genetic testing was not consistent from subject to subject. Only a subset of patients who were found to have one or fewer variants by direct sequencing were subjected to MLPA. In addition, for cases in which two or more pathogenic variants were identified by direct sequencing, no further analyses were performed, and the presence of large deletions may have been missed. Gülin Evinç et al. in Turkey report that children with untreated Phe levels of 240–360 μmol/L are at a higher risk for cognitive and behavioral impairment as compared to healthy children [27]. To evaluate neurodevelopmental outcome, appropriate developmental testing should have been performed in this study.

Based on study findings, we propose the following measures when p.R53H is detected by genotype search about HPA of NBS in Japan. When identifying patients with PKU carrying p.R53H, presence of two other pathogenic variants should be looked for. Whereas, when patients with HPA carrying p.R53H are identified, *p.R53H* should be considered underlying the phenotype. This study revealed that blood Phe levels in patients with HPA carrying p.R53H were continuously below 360 μmol/L without diet therapy. However, we should not determine the follow-up frequency only by genotype. We suggest monthly follow-up at least in their infancy according to their diet change and increase in protein intake. The patients with persistently low Phe levels during infancy may not require the frequent hospital visits and the frequent measurements of blood Phe levels. In summary, we could clarify genotype–phenotype correlations and long-term follow-up data on blood Phe levels in patients with p.R53H and one genotype associated with PKU in the Japanese population. We therefore consider that the findings of our study hold implications in strategically planning appropriate follow-ups for patients with HPA. Future studies should investigate patient-oriented outcomes in the clinical management.

Supplementary Materials: The following are available online at https://www.mdpi.com/2409-515X/7/1/17/s1, Table S1: PAH variations (*n* = 370) found in the study cohort of PKU patients.

Author Contributions: Conceptualization and methodology, all authors; writing—original draft preparation, S.O., H.S., and T.H.; statistical analyses, D.K., S.T., and K.Y.; genetic analyses, S.K., T.S., and N.N. All authors have read and agreed to the published version of the manuscript.

Funding: This work was supported in part by Health and Labor Sciences Research Grant 20316977 (to T.H.), and AMED JP16ek0109050, JP19ek0109276, JP20ek0109482 (to T.H.).

Institutional Review Board Statement: The study was conducted according to the guidelines of the Declaration of Helsinki, and approved by the Institutional Review Board of Osaka City University Graduate School of Medicine (protocol code 3687, 27/02/2017).

Informed Consent Statement: Informed consent was obtained from all subjects or their parents/guardians involved in the study.

Data Availability Statement: The data that support the findings of this study are available from the corresponding author, T.H., upon reasonable request.

Conflicts of Interest: The authors declare no conflict of interest.

References

1. Blau, N.; van Spronsen, F.J.; Levy, H.L. Phenylketonuria. *Lancet* **2010**, *376*, 1417–1427. [CrossRef]
2. Okano, Y.; Eisensmith, R.C.; Güttler, F.; Lichter-Konecki, U.; Konecki, D.S.; Trefz, F.K.; Dasovich, M.; Wang, T.; Henriksen, K.; Lou, H.; et al. Molecular Basis of Phenotypic Heterogeneity in Phenylketonuria. *N. Engl. J. Med.* **1991**, *324*, 1232–1238. [CrossRef]
3. Guldberg, P.; Rey, F.; Zschocke, J.; Romano, V.; François, B.; Michiels, L.; Ullrich, K.; Hoffmann, G.F.; Burgard, P.; Schmidt, H.; et al. A European Multicenter Study of Phenylalanine Hydroxylase Deficiency: Classification of 105 Mutations and a General System for Genotype-Based Prediction of Metabolic Phenotype. *Am. J. Hum. Genet.* **1998**, *63*, 71–79. [CrossRef] [PubMed]
4. Van Wegberg, A.M.J.; Macdonald, A.; Ahring, K.; BéLanger-Quintana, A.; Blau, N.; Bosch, A.M.; Burlina, A.; Campistol, J.; Feillet, F.; Giżewska, M.; et al. The complete European guidelines on phenylketonuria: Diagnosis and treatment. *Orphanet J. Rare Dis.* **2017**, *12*, 1–56. [CrossRef]
5. Camp, K.M.; Parisi, M.A.; Acosta, P.B.; Berry, G.T.; Bilder, D.A.; Blau, N.; Bodamer, O.A.; Brosco, J.P.; Brown, C.S.; Burlina, A.B.; et al. Phenylketonuria Scientific Review Conference: State of the science and future research needs. *Mol. Genet. Metab.* **2014**, *112*, 87–122. [CrossRef]

6. Nagasaki, M.; Yasuda, J.; Katsuoka, F.; Nariai, N.; Kojima, K.; Kawai, Y.; Yamaguchi-Kabata, Y.; Yokozawa, J.; Danjoh, I.; Saito, S.; et al. Rare variant discovery by deep whole-genome sequencing of 1,070 Japanese individuals. *Nat. Commun.* **2015**, *6*, 8018. [CrossRef]
7. Dateki, S.; Watanabe, S.; Nakatomi, A.; Kinoshita, E.; Matsumoto, T.; Yoshiura, K.I.; Moriuchi, H. Genetic background of hyperphenylalaninemia in Nagasaki, Japan. *Pediatr. Int.* **2016**, *58*, 431–433. [CrossRef]
8. Lee, D.H.; Koo, S.K.; Lee, K.-S.; Yeon, Y.-J.; Oh, H.-J.; Kim, S.-W.; Lee, S.-J.; Kim, S.-S.; Lee, J.-E.; Jo, I.; et al. The molecular basis of phenylketonuria in Koreans. *J. Hum. Genet.* **2004**, *49*, 617–621. [CrossRef]
9. Li, N.; He, C.; Li, J.; Tao, J.; Liu, Z.; Zhang, C.; Yuan, Y.; Jiang, H.; Zhu, J.; Deng, Y.; et al. Analysis of the genotype-phenotype correlation in patients with phenylketonuria in mainland China. *Sci. Rep.* **2018**, *8*, 1–7. [CrossRef]
10. Park, Y.S.; Seoung, C.S.; Lee, S.W.; Oh, K.H.; Lee, D.H.; Yim, J. Identification of three novel mutations in Korean phenylketonuria patients: R53H, N207D, and Y325X. *Hum. Mutat.* **1998**, *11*, S121–S122. [CrossRef]
11. Okano, Y.; Kudo, S.; Nishi, Y.; Sakaguchi, T.; Aso, K. Molecular characterization of phenylketonuria and tetrahydrobiopterin-responsive phenylalanine hydroxylase deficiency in Japan. *J. Hum. Genet.* **2011**, *56*, 306–312. [CrossRef]
12. Liang, Y.; Huang, M.-Z.; Cheng, C.-Y.; Chao, H.-K.; Fwu, V.T.; Chiang, S.-H.; Hsiao, K.-J.; Niu, D.-M.; Su, T.-S. The mutation spectrum of the phenylalanine hydroxylase (PAH) gene and associated haplotypes reveal ethnic heterogeneity in the Taiwanese population. *J. Hum. Genet.* **2014**, *59*, 145–152. [CrossRef]
13. Tao, J.; Li, N.; Jia, H.; Liu, Z.; Li, X.; Song, J.; Deng, Y.; Jin, X.; Zhu, J. Correlation between genotype and the tetrahydrobiopterin-responsive phenotype in Chinese patients with phenylketonuria. *Pediatr. Res.* **2015**, *78*, 691–699. [CrossRef]
14. Eisensmith, R.C.; Woo, S.L.C. Molecular basis of phenylketonuria and related hyperphenylalaninemias: Mutations and polymorphisms in the human phenylalanine hydroxylase gene. *Hum. Mutat.* **1992**, *1*, 13–23. [CrossRef] [PubMed]
15. Ellingsen, S.; Knappskog, P.M.; Eiken, H.G. Phenylketonuria splice mutation (EXON6nt-96Ag) masquerading as missense mutation (Y204C). *Hum. Mutat.* **1997**, *9*, 88–90. [CrossRef]
16. Santos, L.L.; Castro-Magalhães, M.; Fonseca, C.G.; Starling, A.L.P.; Januário, J.N.; Aguiar, M.J.B.; Carvalho, M.R.S. PKU in Minas Gerais State, Brazil: Mutation analysis. *Ann. Hum. Genet.* **2008**, *72*, 774–779. [CrossRef]
17. Li, N.; Jia, H.; Liu, Z.; Tao, J.; Chen, S.; Li, X.; Deng, Y.; Jin, X.; Song, J.; Zhang, L.; et al. Molecular characterisation of phenylketonuria in a Chinese mainland population using next-generation sequencing. *Sci. Rep.* **2016**, *5*, 15769. [CrossRef]
18. Hennermann, J.B.; Vetter, B.; Wolf, C.; Windt, E.; Bührdel, P.; Seidel, J.; Mönch, E.; Kulozik, A.E. Phenylketonuria and hyperphenylalaninemia in eastern Germany: A characteristic molecular profile and 15 novel mutations. *Hum Mutat.* **2000**, *15*, 254–260. [CrossRef]
19. Okano, Y.; Asada, M.; Kang, Y.; Nishi, Y.; Hase, Y.; Oura, T.; Isshiki, G. Molecular characterization of phenylketonuria in Japanese patients. *Hum Genet.* **1998**, *103*, 613–618. [CrossRef]
20. Okano, Y.; Hase, Y.; Lee, D.H.; Furuyama, J.I.; Shintaku, H.; Oura, T.; Isshiki, G. Frequency and distribution of phenylketonuric mutations in orientals. *Hum. Mutat.* **1992**, *1*, 216–220. [CrossRef]
21. Koshiba, S.; Motoike, I.; Kojima, K.; Hasegawa, T.; Shirota, M.; Saito, T.; Saigusa, D.; Danjoh, I.; Katsuoka, F.; Ogishima, S.; et al. The structural origin of metabolic quantitative diversity. *Sci. Rep.* **2016**, *6*, 31463. [CrossRef]
22. Choi, R.; Lee, J.; Park, H.D.; Park, J.E.; Kim, Y.H.; Ki, C.S.; Lee, S.Y.; Song, J.; Kim, J.W.; Lee, D.H. Reassessing the significance of the PAH c.158G>A (p.Arg53His) mutation in patients with hyperphenylalaninemia. *J. Pediatr. Endocrinol. Metab.* **2017**, *30*, 1211–1218. [CrossRef]
23. Hillert, A.; Anikster, Y.; Belanger-Quintana, A.; Burlina, A.; Burton, B.K.; Carducci, C.; Chiesa, A.E.; Christodoulou, J.; Đorđević, M.; Blau, N.; et al. The Genetic Landscape and Epidemiology of Phenylketonuria. *Am. J. Hum. Genet.* **2020**, *107*, 234–250. [CrossRef]
24. Blau, N.; Ichinose, H.; Nagatsu, T.; Heizmann, C.W.; Zacchello, F.; Burlina, A.B. A missense mutation in a patient with guanosine triphosphate cyclohydrolase I deficiency missed in the newborn screening program. *J. Pediatr.* **1995**, *126*, 401–405. [CrossRef]
25. Blau, N.; Martinez, A.; Hoffmann, G.F.; Thöny, B. DNAJC12 deficiency: A new strategy in the diagnosis of hyperphenylalaninemias. *Mol. Genet. Metab.* **2018**, *123*, 1–5. [CrossRef]
26. Japanese Society for Inherited Metabolic Disease. *Newborn Screening Clinical Guideline*; Shindan to Chiryo Sha: Tokyo, Japan, 2019; pp. 11–24. (In Japanese)
27. Evinç, S.G.; Pektaş, E.; Foto-Özdemir, D.; Yıldız, Y.; Karaboncuk, Y.; Bilginer-Gürbüz, B.; Dursun, A.; Tokatlı, A.; Coskun, T.; Öktem, F.; et al. Cognitive and behavioral impairment in mild hyperphenylalaninemia. *Turk. J. Pediatr.* **2018**, *60*, 617–624. [CrossRef]

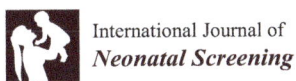

Review

Newborn Screening for Congenital Hypothyroidism in Japan

Kanshi Minamitani

Department of Pediatrics, Teikyo University Chiba Medical Center, Chiba 299-0111, Japan; kminami@med.teikyo-u.ac.jp; Tel.: +81-436-62-1211

Abstract: Congenital hypothyroidism (CH) is the most common preventable cause of intellectual impairment or failure to thrive by early identification and treatment. In Japan, newborn screening programs for CH were introduced in 1979, and the clinical guidelines for newborn screening of CH were developed in 1998, revised in 2014, and are currently undergoing further revision. Newborn screening strategies are designed to detect the elevated levels of thyroid stimulating hormone (TSH) in most areas of Japan, although TSH and free thyroxine (FT4) are often measured simultaneously in some areas. Since 1987, in order not to observe the delayed rise in TSH, additional rescreening of premature neonates and low birth weight infants (<2000 g) at four weeks of life or when their body weight reaches 2500 g has been recommended, despite a normal initial newborn screening. Recently, the actual incidence of CH has doubled to approximately 1:2500 in Japan as in other countries. This increasing incidence is speculated to be mainly due to an increase in the number of mildly affected patients detected by the generalized lowering of TSH screening cutoffs and an increase in the number of preterm or low birth weight neonates at a higher risk of having CH than term infants.

Keywords: newborn screening; lowering of thyroid stimulating hormone screening cutoffs; thyroid dysgenesis; thyroid dyshormonogenesis; transient congenital hypothyroidism; permanent congenital hypothyroidism; delayed rise in TSH; low birth weight

Citation: Minamitani, K. Newborn Screening for Congenital Hypothyroidism in Japan. *Int. J. Neonatal Screen.* **2021**, *7*, 34. https://doi.org/10.3390/ijns7030034

Academic Editor: Ralph Fingerhut

Received: 27 May 2021
Accepted: 23 June 2021
Published: 28 June 2021

Publisher's Note: MDPI stays neutral with regard to jurisdictional claims in published maps and institutional affiliations.

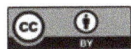

Copyright: © 2021 by the author. Licensee MDPI, Basel, Switzerland. This article is an open access article distributed under the terms and conditions of the Creative Commons Attribution (CC BY) license (https://creativecommons.org/licenses/by/4.0/).

1. Introduction

Since thyroid hormone is indispensable for myelin sheath formation during the fetal, neonatal, and infant periods, dysfunction of thyroid hormone during these periods causes irreversible intelligence impairment. Furthermore, thyroid hormone stimulates growth hormone secretion, insulin-like growth factor 1 production, and bone maturation. Therefore, insufficient thyroid hormone activity can result in failure to thrive and early osteoporosis in adulthood. Primary congenital hypothyroidism (CH) is the most common congenital endocrine disorder caused mainly by thyroid dysgenesis or thyroid dyshormonogenesis. CH can be prevented by early detection and optimal treatment, and newborn screening programs for CH have been introduced in many countries worldwide. In Japan, newborn screening programs for CH started in 1979 and have markedly improved neurologic and health outcomes [1–3]. The present review provides an update on newborn screening programs for CH as well as the treatment and long-term outcomes of CH in Japan.

2. Newborn Screening Programs for CH

Before the development of newborn screening programs for CH, primary CH was mainly diagnosed from clinical symptoms based on a 12-item checklist (persistent jaundice, constipation, umbilical hernia, poor weight gain, xerosis cutis, sluggishness, macroglossia, hoarseness, coldness of limbs, edema, dilation of posterior fontanel, and goiter) [4]. However, because these symptoms are nonspecific in the neonatal period, they were often diagnosed late or overlooked. Newborn screening for CH through an enzyme immunoassay-based thyroid stimulating hormone (TSH) measurement on a filter paper blood spot sample was introduced as a nationwide screening program in 1979, and this method was upgraded to enzyme-linked immunosorbent assay in 1987 [2,5,6]. At present, patients with CH are treated according to the guidelines of mass screening for CH by the Japanese Society for Pediatric Endocrinology and the Japanese Society for Mass Screening, which were developed in 1998 [7] and revised in 2014 [8].

An initial TSH-based screening is performed using a filter paper blood spot sample collected on days 5–7 postpartum. Neonates with a TSH level of 15–30 mIU/L in whole blood on the filter paper blood spot sample are immediately referred to a regional medical facility for closer clinical examination. Neonates with a TSH level of 10–15 mIU/L are retested for TSH using the filter paper blood spot sample. Neonates with a TSH level >10 mIU/L in the retested sample are usually subjected to close examination [8].

Currently, the age of the first visit for close examination of patients ranges from 15.8 to 18 days, with an average of 17.3 days [3].

During close examination in a medical facility, the family history of thyroid disease and mother's history of iodine overload and medication are noted. In Japan, where iodine is abundant, dietary iodine insufficiency is rarely seen. A physical examination is performed mainly based on the abovementioned 12 items of the checklist. Serum TSH, free thyroxine (FT4), free triiodothyronine (FT3), and thyroglobulin levels are measured. The distal femoral epiphyseal ossification center (DFEC) is examined using X-ray, and the thyroid gland is identified using ultrasonography. Thyroid scintigraphy is reliable for the definitive diagnosis of thyroid dysgenesis. However, it is generally not performed in the neonatal period in Japan, probably because it is the only atomic-bombed country in the world.

Treatment is immediately initiated under following conditions: if a case has clinical symptoms, if the appearance of the DFEC is delayed, if the thyroid gland cannot be identified by ultrasonography, or if goiter is found. It is recommended to start treatment if the serum TSH level is $\geq$30 mIU/L or 15–30 mIU/L and the FT4 level is $\leq$15 pmol/L.

If no clinical symptoms are found, the serum FT4 level is within the normal range, and the TSH level is <15 mIU/L, a thyroid function test should be performed again. If the serum TSH level is >10 mIU/L at 3–4 weeks after birth, treatment initiation should be considered. It has been suggested that infants with a TSH level of $\geq$10 mIU/L at <6 months after birth and $\geq$5 mIU/L at 12 months after birth should be followed up carefully and treated.

3. Incidence of CH in Japan

Prior to the introduction of newborn screening for CH, the incidence of primary CH was 1:7400 [1]. However, once screening was started, the incidence increased to 1:3000 to 4000 since the 1990s and then to 1:2000 to 2500 since the 2000s [5]. The possible reasons for this increase include an increase in the number of mildly affected patients detected by the generalized lowering of TSH screening cutoffs and an increase in the number of preterm or low birth weight neonates at a higher risk of having CH than term infants, as well as epigenetic factors and changes in iodine intake and dietary habits [9].

The percentage of regions with the positive criterion of a TSH level of $\leq$30 mIU/L in whole blood on the filter paper blood spot sample doubled from 43.1% in 1993 to 89.4% in 2008 [10]. Therefore, the identification of an additional mild form of CH with gland-in-situ is thought to be responsible for the increase in CH incidence.

Preterm or low birth weight neonates are at a higher risk of having CH than term infants. In Japan, recent dramatic advances in neonatal care have led to an increase in the percentage of low birth weight neonates in Japan, i.e., from 5.2% in 1975 to 9.4% in 2017 [11]. However, there are no reports on the actual incidence of CH in low birth weight neonates in Japan.

4. Epidemiology of CH in Japan

Iodine deficiency is rare in Japan, which is originally an iodine-sufficient area. According to data from 1989, CH was caused by thyroid dysgenesis in 84% of cases (ectopic thyroid gland in 60% and athyreosis/hypoplasia of the thyroid gland in 24%) and by intrinsic defects of thyroid hormone synthesis (dyshormonogenesis) in the remaining 16% cases [12]. However, several recent studies using lower cutoff points for TSH levels have reported an increased diagnosis of cases with gland-in-situ. In a 2008 Japanese study, 54% of primary CH cases were caused by thyroid dysgenesis (ectopic thyroid gland in 37% and athyreosis/hypoplasia of the thyroid gland in 17%) and the remaining 46% of CH cases occurred due to dyshormonogenesis [13].

A comprehensive genetic analysis identifies genetic abnormalities in 20% of Japanese patients [14–18]. Mutations in the DUOX2 gene are particularly common, identified in approximately 20% cases of dyshormonogenesis. In contrast, in thyroid dysgenesis, genetic mutations can only be identified in 5–10% of patients.

Currently, the National Center for Child Health and Development (Tokyo, Japan) analyzes genetic mutations in CH-associated genes, including DUOX2, DUOXA2, FOXE1, GLIS3, IGSF1, IYD, NKX2-1, PAX8, SECISBP2, SLC26A4, SLC5A5, TG, THRA, THRB, TPO, TRH, TRHR, TSHB, and TSHR, using next-generation sequencing methods.

5. CH in Low Birth Weight Neonates

Premature and low birth weight neonates may present with hypothyroxinemia without an increase in the TSH level through a variety of mechanisms, including the hypothalamic–pituitary–thyroid axis immaturity, nonthyroidal illness, dopamine administration, high-dose steroid therapy, undernutrition, and exchange transfusion [19]. A delayed rise in TSH is a condition in which although the TSH level is below the cutoff point at initial screening, it increases later. A delayed rise in TSH is particularly common in low birth weight infants. A retrospective single-center matched case-control study shows that the percentage of small-for-gestational age infants was significantly higher in the delayed TSH rise group (71%) than in the comparison group (25%) [20]. In order not to overlook this pattern of delayed rise in TSH, since 1987, additional rescreening of premature neonates and low birth weight infants (<2000 g) at four weeks of life, when their body weight reaches 2500 g, or at discharge from the hospital is recommended, despite a normal initial newborn screening [21,22].

More than 50% of low birth weight infants before 30 weeks of gestational age manifest a temporary pattern of low levels of FT4 and normal or low levels of TSH termed 'transient hypothyroxinemia of prematurity' (THOP), due to the immaturity of the hypothalamic-pituitary-thyroid axis, iodine deficiency, the withdrawal of maternal placenta FT4 transfer, nonthyroidal illness and exposure to some medications. The more premature the infants are, the more severely the thyroxine is reduced. Many studies have shown that levothyroxine sodium (LT4) has a poor effect on severe hypothyroxinemia [23–25], and the administration of LT4 to premature infants in Japan has been suggested to cause late onset circulatory collapse [26,27]. Infants with THOP should not be treated with LT4.

6. Treatment of CH

The Japanese Guidelines classify serum FT4 level <5, 5 to <10, and 10 to <15 pmol/L as indicating most severe, severe, and moderate cases, respectively, taking into consideration the consensus guidelines of the European Society for Pediatric Endocrinology [28].

Treatment starts with the administration of 10 μg/kg/day LT4 in powder form once daily before breakfast. In most severe cases, treatment starts with a dose of 12–15 μg/kg/day LT4. Infants with subclinical CH can be treated with 3–5 μg/kg/day LT4 because they often become hyperthyroid when given 10 μg/kg/day LT4 [8].

The target for serum FT4 levels should be >50% of the reference range by age. The target for TSH level should be the reference range by age. A follow-up is required at one, two, and four weeks after the start of LT4 treatment, at one-month intervals until one year of age, and then at 3–4-month intervals until the adult stage.

7. Re-Evaluation

A re-evaluation or definitive diagnosis should be made for the patients with CH after the age of three years, including the differentiation of transient from persistent CH [8]. After four weeks of LT4 withdrawal, a ^{123}I thyroid scintigram, ^{123}I uptake rate, saliva/serum iodine ratio, perchlorate discharge test, thyroid function tests (TSH, FT4, FT3, and thyroglobulin), and thyroid ultrasonography are performed to diagnose athyreosis, hypoplasia, ectopic thyroid gland, hormone organification defect, and iodine concentration deficiency. If no abnormalities are detected upon these examinations, the patient is diagnosed with transient hypothyroidism. Infants treated with less than 1.25 µg/kg/day LT4 at three years of age are more likely to have transient CH [29,30]. In addition, infants who do not require an increase in LT4 dose after three years of age are more likely to have transient CH [31].

8. Psychomotor Development

Prior to newborn screening for CH, only 19.8% of infants with CH received treatment at an age of less than three months. Therefore, even after treatment, 43% of the patients showed mental retardation with IQ levels below 75, 33.3% of the patients showed IQ levels over 90, and two thirds of the patients were mentally retarded, including those on the borderline [32].

In early newborn screening, the recommended initial dose of LT4 was 5–8 µg/kg/day, and the initiation of treatment was often delayed until 4–5 weeks after birth. The patients with CH had an IQ that was lower by 6–20 points in comparison with controls, and the prognosis was particularly poor in severe children with a blood T4 level < 5 µg/dL at their initial visit. The mean IQ in the first nationwide survey in 1991 was 97.5 ± 14.8 ($n = 81$) [33] and that in the second survey in 1994 was 99.9 ± 13.7 ($n = 151$) [34].

Since the late 1990s, infants with CH have been treated with an initial dose of 10–15 µg/kg/day LT4, with treatment starting within two weeks after birth [35]. In the nationwide follow-up survey of CH children in 2003 [36], the DQ/IQ at 1–5 years of age was good, ranging from 104.1 to 107.3. Serious intellectual disability due to CH has almost been eradicated. However, children with severe hypothyroidism, such as athyreosis, during pregnancy presented with significantly lower IQ levels than those with other types of CH [37]. Furthermore, patients with severe CH also have cognitive, behavioral, and attention deficits in adolescence and adulthood [35,36].

9. Growth, Puberty, Body Composition, and Quality of Life

Prior to newborn screening for CH, while the frequency of children with a high degree of short stature equal to or less than −3 SD decreased from 45% to 11.8% after LT4 treatment, the frequency of children with a short stature equal to or less than −2 SD represented approximately 30% [32].

A report analyzing the height and body weight of 2341 patients with CH (1030 males and 1311 females) detected neither short stature nor obesity, but normal growth and constitution through a registration in the Medical Aid Program for Chronic Pediatric Disease of Specified Categories in 2002 [38]. A follow-up study in 2006 reported that the patients with CH had a nearly normal physique, with a height of 162.9 ± 8.4 cm and body weight of 60.8 ± 14.3 kg for male adults, height of 157.3 ± 5.2 cm and body weight of 52.4 ± 7.4 kg for female adults, and BMI of approximately 21.1 ± 3.0 for both males and females [39]. A report from Kanagawa shows no significant difference in adolescent growth patterns and adult height between patients with CH and healthy individuals, and no significant correlation between adult height and severity of hypothyroidism or the age of starting treatment was observed [40]. Some reports suggest that, even with good control, puberty tends to be earlier in girls with CH, judging from the age at menarche [41,42].

Patients in whom CH was detected shortly after the introduction of newborn screening have already finished compulsory education and reached the age for employment or marriage. The long-term quality of life (QOL) condition of these patients has been reported [39,41]. Regarding the employment status of these patients, full time employees represent 27% of patients, part-time employees represent 10%, unemployed represent 8%, married and unemployed represent 6%, students represent 43%, and others represent 6%, with no difference in employment status compared with the general population of the same generation. Patients with CH show no differences in academic backgrounds for employees and the unemployed compared with those of the general population, as 15% of patients graduated from university/college, 7% dropped out from university/college, 22% graduated from vocational school or junior college, 41% graduated from high school, 4% dropped out from high school, and 11% graduated from junior high school. In terms of marital status, 8% of the patients with CH are married. In Japan, more than 90% of all households purchase life insurance. Life insurance aims to cover the loss associated with life, accidents, and sickness and also meets various needs, such as savings and post-retirement security, but people with underlying conditions are often refused enrollment by life insurance companies. Among patients with CH, 46% have purchased life insurance and 65% of them applied for their insurance without declaring their disease [39].

10. Summary

Newborn screening for CH markedly improves the long-term intellectual outcome, physical growth, and QOL of patients with CH.

The incidence of CH is increasing every year. It is important to minimize the damage of hypothyroidism and further improve the outcomes by setting appropriate cutoff values, appropriate initial therapeutic doses, and appropriate treatment for mild CH and low birth weight infants.

Given that some patients with CH are anxious about explaining their disease to their spouses and the inheritance of the disease, proper counseling needs to be provided based on genetic diagnosis. In addition, it is becoming apparent that patients have various issues, including their transition from the pediatric to adult clinic, purchase of life insurance, and burden of medical expenses.

Funding: This research received no external funding.

Data Availability Statement: No new data were created or analyzed in this study. Data sharing is not applicable to this article.

Conflicts of Interest: The author declares no conflict of interest.

References

1. Nakajima, H.; Satoh, K.; Inomata, H.; Matsuura, N.; Okaniwa, S.; Igarashi, H.; Yokoyama, S.; Okabe, I.; Yamaguchi, S.; Tsuchiya, Y.; et al. National study of mental development of patients with congenital hypothyroidism disclosed by neonatal mass screening. *J. Jpn. Pediatr. Soc.* **1989**, *93*, 2011–2016. (In Japanese)
2. Niimi, H. Neonatal screening for congenital hypothyrodism and hyperthyrotropinemia without hypothyroxinemia. *Clin. Pediatr. Endocrinol.* **1994**, *3*, 73–77. [CrossRef]
3. Inomata, H.; Aoki, K. National survey of congenital hypothyroidism detected by neonatal mass screening (1994–1999). *Jpn. J. Mass Screen.* **2003**, *13*, 27–32. (In Japanese)
4. Nakajima, H. Congenital hypothyroidism. In *Handbook of Neonatal Screening*; Naruse, H., Matsuda, I., Eds.; Nankodo Co., Ltd.: Tokyo, Japan, 1989; pp. 100–110. (In Japanese)
5. Minamitani, K.; Inomata, H. Neonatal screening for congenital hypothyroidism in Japan. *Pediatr. Endocrinol. Rev.* **2012**, *10* (Suppl. 1), 79–88.
6. Fukushi, M. Screening for congenital hypothyroidism. *Lab. Sci. Neonatal Mass Screen.* **2000**, *19*, 12–19. (In Japanese)
7. Inomata, H.; Matsuura, N.; Tachibana, K.; Kusuda, S.; Fukushi, M.; Umehashi, H.; Suwa, S.; Niimi, H.; Fujieda, K.; Working Group on Congenital Hypothyroidism of the Japanese Society for Pediatric Endocrinology and the Japanese Society for Mass-screening. Guideline for neonatal mass-screening for congenital hypothyroidism (1998). *Clin. Pediatr. Endocrinol.* **1999**, *8*, 1–55. [CrossRef]
8. Mass Screening Committee, Japanese Society for Pediatric Endocrinology; Japanese Society for Mass Screening; Nagasaki, K.; Minamitani, K.; Anzo, M.; Adachi, M.; Ishii, T.; Onigata, K.; Kusuda, S.; Harada, S.; et al. Guidelines for mass screening of congenital hypothyroidism (2014 version). *Clin. Pediatr. Endocrinol.* **2015**, *24*, 107–133. [PubMed]
9. Wassner, A.J.; Brown, R.S. Congenital hypothyroidism: Recent advances. *Curr. Opin. Endocrinol. Diabetes Obes.* **2015**, *22*, 407–412. [CrossRef] [PubMed]
10. Minamitani, K.; Sugihara, S.; Inomata, H.; Harada, S. Re-evaluation of neonatal screening system for congenital hypothyroidism in Japan. *Jpn. J. Mass Screen.* **2009**, *19*, 51–57. (In Japanese)
11. Director-General for Statistics and Information Policy, Ministry of Health, Labour and Welfare. Vital Statistics in Japan. Available online: https://www.mhlw.go.jp/toukei/list/dl/81-1a2.pdf (accessed on 14 May 2021). (In Japanese).
12. Sato, H.; Nakajima, H. The 7th and 8th national studies of the patients with congenital hypothyroidism and its related diseases found on neonatal screening. *J. Jpn. Pediatr. Soc.* **1989**, *93*, 1152–1158. (In Japanese)

13. Minamitani, K.; Harada, S.; Nagasaki, K.; Tajima, T. *Etiology of Congenital Hypothyroidism Analyzed from Follow-Up Surveys in Chiba, Hokkaido, and Niigata*; Annual Report; Research on the Construction and Analysis of Databases on Child Health and Development and Their Information Provision from Health Labour Sciences Research Grant; The Ministry of Health Labour and Welfare: Tokyo, Japan, 2009; pp. 70–74.
14. Narumi, S.; Muroya, K.; Asakura, Y.; Adachi, M.; Hasegawa, T. Transcription factor mutations and congenital hypothyroidism: Systematic genetic screening of a population-based cohort of Japanese patients. *J. Clin. Endocrinol. Metab.* **2010**, *95*, 1981–1985. [CrossRef]
15. Narumi, S.; Muroya, K.; Asakura, Y.; Aachi, M.; Hasegawa, T. Molecular basis of thyroid dyshormonogenesis: Genetic screening in population-based Japanese patients. *J. Clin. Endocrinol. Metab.* **2011**, *96*, E1838–E1842. [CrossRef]
16. Yamaguchi, T.; Nakamura, A.; Nakayama, K.; Hishimura, N.; Morikawa, S.; Ishizu, K.; Tajima, T. Targeted next-generation sequencing for congenital hypothyroidism with positive neonatal TSH screening. *J. Clin. Endocrinol. Metab.* **2020**, *105*, dgaa308. [CrossRef]
17. Tanaka, T.; Aoyama, K.; Suzuki, A.; Saitoh, S.; Mizuno, H. Clinical and genetic investigation of 136 Japanese patients with congenital hypothyroidism. *J. Pediatr. Endocrinol. Metab.* **2020**, *33*, 691–701. [CrossRef] [PubMed]
18. Matsuo, K.; Tanahashi, Y.; Mukai, T.; Suzuki, S.; Tajima, T.; Azuma, H.; Fujieda, K. High prevalence of DUOX2 mutations in Japanese patients with permanent congenital hypothyroidism or transient hypothyroidism. *J. Pediatr. Endocrinol. Metab.* **2016**, *29*, 807–812. [CrossRef] [PubMed]
19. Cherella, C.E.; Wassner, A.J. Update on congenital hypothyroidism. *Curr. Opin. Endocrinol. Diabetes Obes.* **2020**, *27*, 63–69. [CrossRef] [PubMed]
20. Uchiyama, A.; Watanabe, H.; Nakanishi, H.; Totsu, S. Small for gestational age is a risk factor for the development of delayed thyrotropin elevation in infants weighing less than 2000 g. *Clin. Endocrinol.* **2018**, *89*, 431–436. [CrossRef]
21. Fukushi, M. Blood sampling of premature baby in newborn screening. *Rep. Found. Metab. Screen.* **1987**, *10*, 29. (In Japanese)
22. Inomata, H.; Nakajima, H.; Aoki, K.; Tchibana, K.; Kuroda, Y. Thirty five cases with congenital primary hypothyroidism undetected by neonatal screening in nation-wide survey. *Clin. Endocrinol.* **2001**, *49*, 1141–1145. (In Japanese)
23. Chowdhry, P.; Scanlon, J.W.; Auerbach, R.; Abbassi, V. Results of controlled double blind study of thyroid replacement in very low-birth-weight premature infants with hypothyroxinemia. *Pediatrics* **1984**, *73*, 301–305. [PubMed]
24. Smith, L.M.; Leake, R.D.; Berman, N.; Villanueva, S.; Brasel, J.A. Postnatal thyroxine supplementation in infants less than 32 weeks' gestation: Effects on pulmonary morbidity. *J. Perinatol.* **2000**, *20*, 427–431. [CrossRef] [PubMed]
25. van Wassenaer, A.G.; Kok, J.H.; de Vijlder, J.J.; Briët, J.M.; Smit, B.J.; Tamminga, P.; van Baar, A.; Dekker, F.W.; Vulsma, T. Effects of thyroxine supplementation on neurologic development in infants born at less than 30 weeks' gestation. *N. Engl. J. Med.* **1997**, *336*, 21–26. [CrossRef]
26. Yagasaki, H.; Kobayashi, K.; Nemoto, A.; Naito, A.; Sugita, K.; Ohyama, K. Late-onset circulatory dysfunction after thyroid hormone treatment in an extremely low birth weight infant. *J. Pediatr. Endocrinol. Metab.* **2010**, *23*, 153–158. [CrossRef]
27. Kawai, M.; Kusuda, S.; Cho, K.; Horikawa, R.; Takizawa, F.; Ono, M.; Hattori, T.; Oshiro, M. Nationwide surveillance of circulatory collapse associated with levothyroxine administration in very-low-birth weight infants in Japan. *Pediatr. Int.* **2012**, *54*, 177–181. [CrossRef]
28. van Trotsenburg, P.; Stoupa, A.; Léger, J.; Rohrer, T.; Peters, C.; Fugazzola, L.; Cassio, A.; Heinrichs, C.; Beauloye, V.; Pohlenz, J.; et al. Congenital hypothyroidism: A 2020–2021 consensus guidelines update—An ENDO-European Reference Network Initiative endorsed by the European Society for Pediatric Endocrinology and the European Society for Endocrinology. *Thyroid* **2021**, *31*, 387–419. [CrossRef]
29. Itonaga, T.; Higuchi, S.; Shimura, K.; Nagasaki, K.; Satoh, M.; Takubo, N.; Takahashi, I.; Sawada, H.; Hasegawa, Y. Levothyroxine dosage as predictor of permanent and transient congenital hypothyroidism: A multicenter retrospective study in Japan. *Horm. Res. Paediatr.* **2019**, *92*, 45–51. [CrossRef]
30. Higuchi, S.; Hasegawa, Y. Levothyroxine dosages less than 2.4 μg/kg/day at 1 year and 1.3 μg/kg/day at 3 years of age may predict transient congenital hypothyroidism. *Clin. Pediatr. Endocrinol.* **2019**, *28*, 127–133. [CrossRef] [PubMed]
31. Yamamura, H.; Kokumai, T.; Furuya, A.; Suzuki, S.; Tanahashi, Y.; Azuma, H. Increase in doses of levothyroxine at the age of 3 years and above is useful for distinguishing transient and permanent congenital hypothyroidism. *Clin. Pediatr. Endocrinol.* **2020**, *29*, 143–149. [CrossRef] [PubMed]
32. Nakajima, H.; Makino, S. Retrospective analysis of congenital hypothyroidism prior to neonatal screening in Japan. *Shonika* **1980**, *21*, 65–71. (In Japanese)
33. Inomata, H.; Nakajima, H.; Sato, H. National study of mental development of patients with congenital hypothyroidism detected by neonatal screening in Japan. Reevaluation of IQ scores with WISC-R revised in 1989. *J. Jpn. Pediatr. Soc.* **1991**, *95*, 2336–2338. (In Japanese)
34. Inomata, H.; Nakajima, H.; Sato, H.; Ohnishi, H.; Niimi, H. Mental development in patients with congenital hypothyroidism detected by neonatal screening in Japan. Results of the second and total nationwide studies. *J. Jpn. Pediatr. Soc.* **1994**, *98*, 33–38. (In Japanese)
35. Inomata, H.; Kuroda, Y. *Mental Development of Patients with Congenital Hypothyroidism Detected by Neonatal Mass Screening for Congenital Hypothyroidism*; The Third Nationwide Study; The Reports of Health Sciences Research Grants (Research on Children and Families); The Ministry of Health Labour and Welfare: Tokyo, Japan, 2001; pp. 487–489. (In Japanese)

36. Inomata, H.; Aoki, K. Nation-wide follow-up results of neonatal mass-screening for congenital hypothyroidism in the year of 1994–1999. *Jpn. J. Mass Screen.* **2003**, *13*, 27–32. (In Japanese)
37. Minamitani, K.; Inomata, H. Congenital hypothyroidism: Long-term outcome. *Clin. Endocrinol.* **2008**, *56*, 905–913. (In Japanese)
38. Sato, H.; Sasaki, N.; Aoki, K.; Kuroda, Y.; Kato, T. Growth of patients with congenital hypothyroidism detected by neonatal screening in Japan. *Pediatr. Int.* **2007**, *49*, 443–446. [CrossRef] [PubMed]
39. Sato, H.; Nakamura, N.; Harada, S.; Kakee, N.; Sasaki, N. Quality of life of young adults with congenital hypothyroidism. *Pediatr. Int.* **2009**, *51*, 126–131. [CrossRef] [PubMed]
40. Adachi, M.; Asakura, Y.; Tachibana, K. Final height and pubertal growth in Japanese patients with congenital hypothyroidism detected by neonatal screening. *Acta Paediatr.* **2003**, *92*, 698–703. [CrossRef]
41. Inomata, H.; Minagawa, M.; Watanabe, T.; Ohnishi, H.; Shimohashi, K.; Kazukawa, I. *Long-Term Outcome (Scholastic Performance and Working Rate) of Patients Finishing Their Compulsory Education with Congenital Hypothyroidism Detected by Neonatal Screening in Chiba*; The Reports of Health Sciences Research Grants (Research on Child and Families); The Ministry of Health Labour and Welfare: Tokyo, Japan, 2003; pp. 37–39. (In Japanese)
42. Asami, T.; Kikuchi, T.; Kamimura, T.; Kinoshita, S.; Uchiyama, M. Precocious puberty in a girl with congenital hypothyroidism receiving continuous L-thyroxine-replacement therapy. *Pediatr. Int.* **2001**, *43*, 87–90. [CrossRef] [PubMed]

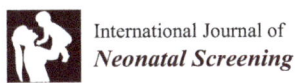

Article

Re-Evaluation of the Prevalence of Permanent Congenital Hypothyroidism in Niigata, Japan: A Retrospective Study

Keisuke Nagasaki [1,*], Hidetoshi Sato [1], Sunao Sasaki [1], Hiromi Nyuzuki [1], Nao Shibata [1], Kentaro Sawano [1], Shota Hiroshima [1] and Tadashi Asami [2]

[1] Department of Homeostatic Regulation and Development, Division of Pediatrics, Niigata University Graduate School of Medical and Dental Sciences, Niigata 951-8510, Japan; totsutotsu0118@gmail.com (H.S.); sunaoenari@gmail.com (S.S.); nyuzuki@med.niigata-u.ac.jp (H.N.); shibata8400@gmail.com (N.S.); sawano@med.niigata-u.ac.jp (K.S.); sho980522@gmail.com (S.H.)

[2] Department of Pediatrics, Nagaoka Institute for Severely Handicapped Children, Nagaoka 940-2135, Japan; tasami@n-seiryo.ac.jp

* Correspondence: nagasaki@med.niigata-u.ac.jp; Tel.: +81-25-227-2222

Abstract: Although newborn screening (NBS) for congenital hypothyroidism (CH) in Japan started more than 40 years ago, the prevalence of CH remains unclear. Prevalence estimations among NBS-positive CH individuals include those with transient hypothyroidism and transient hyperthyrotropinemia, and re-evaluation with increasing age is necessary to clarify the actual incidence. Thus, we re-evaluated the incidence of permanent CH. Of the 106,114 patients who underwent NBS in the Niigata Prefecture, Japan, between April 2002 and March 2006, 116 were examined further due to high thyroid-stimulating hormone levels (>8 mIU/L) and were included in the study. We retrospectively evaluated their levothyroxine sodium (LT4) replacement therapy status from the first visit to 15 years of age. Of the 116 NBS-positive patients, 105 (91%) were initially examined in our department. Of these, 72 (69%) started LT4 replacement therapy on the first visit. Subsequently, 27 patients continued LT4 replacement until 15 years of age after multiple re-evaluations. The prevalence of permanent CH in the Niigata Prefecture during this period was 1 in 2500–3500 children. Ultimately, 62.5% of patients on LT4 replacement discontinued treatment by 15 years of age. This is the first study to clarify the true prevalence of permanent CH in Japan.

Keywords: congenital hypothyroidism; newborn screening; Japan; re-evaluations; prevalence

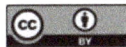

1. Introduction

In Japan, newborn screening (NBS) for congenital hypothyroidism (CH) was initiated in 1979. The prevalence of CH in Japan was initially estimated at 1 in 7400 newborns prior to the commencement of the NBS [1]. National survey results after starting NBS indicated that the prevalence of CH in Japan was 1 in 1600–2500 children since the 2000s [1,2]. CH detected by NBS has been reported in various countries worldwide, but the incidence varies from 1 in 1000 to 1 in 6000 children [3]. Recently, reports have indicated that the prevalence of CH detected by NBS is increasing due to lower thyroid-stimulating hormone (TSH) cut-off values, racial composition changes, and an increase in the number of preterm or low-birthweight infants [3–5].

NBS-positive individuals present with transient hypothyroidism and transient hyperthyrotropinemia [6], and re-evaluation with increasing age is necessary to differentiate between these conditions and determine the actual incidence of CH. Permanent CH prevalence, excluding transient hypothyroidism, has not been clarified in Japan, which prompted our retrospective re-evaluation. To clarify the true prevalence of permanent CH in Niigata, Japan, we re-evaluated the patients who were NBS-positive for CH to determine the permanent CH prevalence based on the levothyroxine sodium (LT4) replacement status.

2. Materials and Methods

This was a single-institution retrospective cohort study. We retrospectively reviewed the LT4 replacement therapy status from the first visit after birth to 15 years of age. In this study, patients on LT4 replacement were defined as CH patients.

2.1. NBS Method in the Niigata Prefecture

Blood samples were collected on filter paper within the first 4 to 7 postnatal days, and the TSH level in the filter paper sample was measured using an enzyme-linked immunosorbent assay (TSH: Enzaplate N-TSH, Bayer Co., Tokyo, Japan). All CH screening tests were centralized at the Niigata Health Laboratory Center.

If the initial TSH level was between 8 and 30 mU/L, a second specimen was evaluated. If the TSH level in the second specimen was also greater than 8 mU/L, a confirmatory test was performed within 30 days of birth at the patient's medical institution. If the initial TSH level was more than 30 mU/L, a confirmatory test was performed within 14 days of birth at the patient's medical institution. Serum-free T4 (FT4), free T3 (FT3), and TSH levels were measured, and the thyroid morphology was evaluated by ultrasonography at the patient's medical institution.

The included patients comprised 116 newborns who tested positive for high TSH levels among the 106,114 newborns who underwent NBS in the Niigata Prefecture, Japan, between April 2002 and March 2006. Patients who had been initially examined at other hospitals were excluded.

2.2. Re-Evaluations at Ages 2–4 Years

Patients with a eutopic thyroid gland who underwent LT4 replacement therapy and remained euthyroid without LT4 dose increments after 12 months of age were re-evaluated by discontinuing LT4 for 4 weeks and performing thyroid function tests.

2.3. Etiological Diagnosis Determination for CH after 5 Years of Age

The methods are detailed in previous studies [7]. To summarize, after discontinuing LT4 replacement therapy, several tests (such as thyroid function test, thyrotropin-releasing hormone stimulation, ^{123}I scintigraphy and radioactive iodine uptake (RAIU), saliva-to-plasma radioiodine ratio, and perchlorate discharge (if the RAIU was 20% or more)) and thyroid ultrasonography were performed.

2.4. Re-Evaluations at Final Height

Patients with a eutopic thyroid gland who underwent LT4 replacement therapy and remained euthyroid after achieving their final height were re-evaluated by discontinuing LT4 for 4 weeks to confirm thyroid function.

2.5. Criteria for Beginning and Discontinuing LT4 Replacement Therapy

The criteria for beginning LT4 were a serum TSH level of 10–15 mU/L or higher at the time of the initial visit, persistent TSH level of $\geq$10 mU/L after the age of 3–6 months, or a persistent TSH level of $\geq$5 mU/L after the age of 1 year. The discontinuation criterion was a serum TSH level of <5 mU/L without LT4 replacement therapy, which was restarted if the TSH level remained above the 5–10 mU/L range.

2.6. Primary and Secondary Outcomes

The primary outcome was the prevalence of permanent CH detected by NBS, and the secondary outcome was the prevalence of transient CH among patients with CH who received LT4 replacement. This study was approved by the Niigata University Ethics Committee. We have published information related to the content of the research on the hospital's homepage. The patients and their parents were informed of their right to refuse access to their medical records for use in the study.

3. Results

The background characteristics of the subjects are listed in Table 1. Fifteen percent of the NBS-positive infants had a low birthweight. Of the 116 NBS-positive subjects with high TSH levels, 105 (91%) were evaluated at our hospital (Figure 1). Therefore, this study is based on a population base of 106,114 × 91% (i.e., 96,000 newborns). The LT4 replacement status for each age group is shown in Figure 2. Of these, 73 patients (69%) were initiated on LT4 at their first visit, while 32 (31%) were left initially untreated; 10 of the latter had persistent mildly elevated TSH levels and were initiated on LT4 by the age of 1 year. Thus, 73 out of 87 patients (84%) were treated with LT4 for 2 years, excluding those who were transferred or those for whom the follow-up had ended.

Table 1. Subject backgrounds.

Sex (n)	Male (54), Female (62)
NBS-positive timing (n)	First examination (28), second examination (88)
Whole blood TSH level in filter paper at NBS **	10.5 (9.8–31.3) mIU/L
Birth weight (BW); mean ± SD (range)	2830 ± 664 g (424–3916)
BW < 2500 g; n (%)	18 (15.5%)
BW < 1500 g; n (%)	8 (6.9%)
Thyroid morphology * (n)	Ectopic (7), hypoplasia (10), enlarged (7), eutopic (81)

n, number of patients; NBS, newborn screening; * Data from 105 patients who underwent detailed examinations at our hospital; ** Data are shown as median (interquartile range).

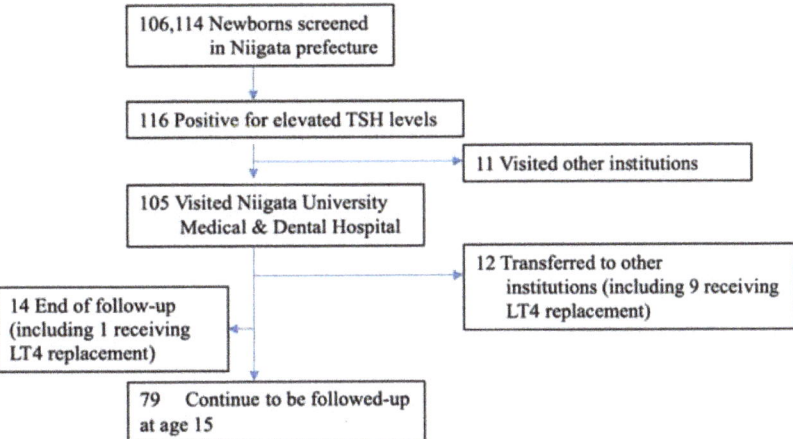

Figure 1. Enrollment of the study subjects. Between April 2002 and March 2006, a total of 106,114 newborns were screened for CH in Niigata prefecture, and 116 were referred to pediatric endocrinologists. We evaluated 105 subjects (90.5%). Eleven patients did not visit our hospital due to reasons such as hospitalization in the neonatal intensive care unit. Fourteen patients (including 1 patient who died after cardiac surgery while on LT4 replacement) with normal thyroid function at the first visit, transient hypothyroidism, or transient hyperthyrotropinemia did not receive further follow-up. Twelve patients, including 9 on LT4 replacement, were transferred to another hospital. At the age of 15, 79 patients were being followed up.

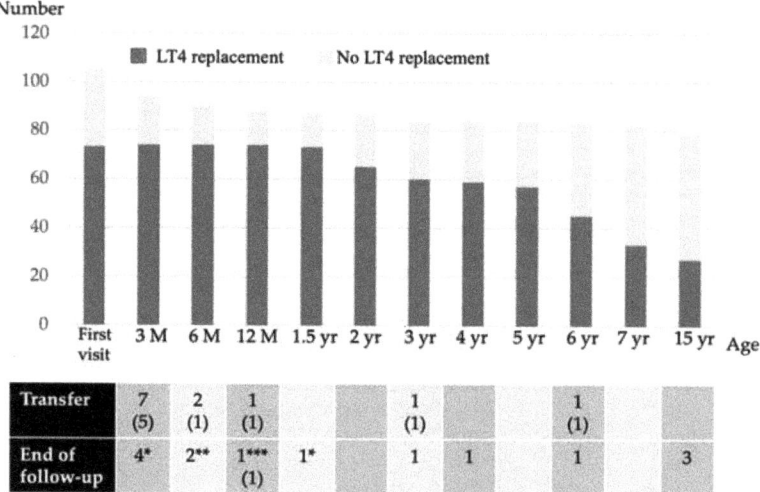

Figure 2. The LT4 replacement status of each age group. M, month; yr, years; (*n*), the number in both parenthesis indicates the number of patients receiving LT4 replacement; * transient hyperthyrotropinemia due to maternal antithyroid drugs or blocking TSH receptor antibody; ** thyroid function was normal from the first visit and the follow-up ended; *** the patient died after cardiac surgery.

Among patients aged between 2 and 5 years, 55 patients were re-evaluated and 16 discontinued LT4 replacement therapy. Consequently, 57 patients were on LT4 replacement therapy at the age of 5 years; of these, 52 patients were diagnosed etiologically with CH at the age of 5–7 years. LT4 replacement was discontinued in 24 patients, and 33 patients were continued on LT4 after the CH etiological diagnosis.

At the re-evaluation conducted after reaching final height, six patients discontinued LT4 replacement therapy, and at 15 years of age, 27 of the 79 patients (34%) who were followed up were receiving LT4 replacement therapy.

3.1. Permanent CH Prevalence

In addition to the 27 patients receiving LT4 replacement at 15 years of age, 10 patients were transferred or died while on LT4 replacement therapy. Thus, the number of patients with permanent CH from April 2002 to March 2006 ranged from 27 to 37, and the permanent CH prevalence was 1 in 2500–3500 children.

3.2. Transient CH Prevalence

Of the 74 patients who received LT4 replacement at 1 year of age, LT4 was discontinued in 46 patients by the age of 15 years, suggesting transient CH. There were 13 NBS-positive infants with an elevated TSH level and a birthweight of less than 2500 g who were examined at our hospital; 11 were initiated on LT4 replacement therapy, 3 were transferred to other hospitals, and 8 discontinued LT4 by the age of 15 years. Thus, the number of patients with transient CH or transient hyperthyrotropinemia ranged from 46 to 56, and the transient CH or transient hyperthyrotropinemia prevalence was 1 in 1700–2100 children.

4. Discussion

In this study, the re-evaluated prevalence of permanent CH was 1 in 2500–3500 children. Approximately 60% of the patients who received LT4 replacement therapy had transient CH or transient hyperthyrotropinemia and discontinued LT4 replacement therapy.

The CH prevalence reported worldwide is likely to include patients with transient hypothyroidism. In our study, when a patient with CH was defined as a patient on LT4 replacement therapy, the CH prevalence was approximately 1 in 1300 children at the time of the first visit after birth, 1 in 1200 children at 1 year of age, and 1 in 1500 children at 5 years of age. The prevalence of CH at 1 year of age increased from the first visit due to the inclusion of patients who started LT4 replacement in early infancy without LT4 replacement at the initial diagnosis, i.e., persistent mild hyperthyrotropinemia. Therefore, when discussing CH prevalence, it is difficult to compare without considering the timing (i.e., age) of the incidences.

Reports indicate that the frequency of transient CH has increased, likely because of lower TSH level cut-off values. The incidence of transient CH in North America is approximately 5% to 10% of the NBS-positive children with CH [8]; however, recent reports indicate that 40% to 53% of the NBS-positive children with CH actually have transient CH [9,10]. Only one-third of patients with CH and eutopic thyroid gland needed to continue LT4 replacement after re-evaluation at the age of 3 to 6 [11]. In our study, approximately 60% of the 74 patients on LT4 replacement therapy at the age of 1 year discontinued it by the age of 15 years. Thus, the TSH cut-off value of 8 mU/L does include a certain number of patients with transient hypothyroidism. Even if LT4 replacement cannot be discontinued by 5 years of age, some patients may be able to discontinue LT4 thereafter and should be re-evaluated for transient CH at the appropriate period.

Increasing numbers of low birthweight and preterm infants may also be associated with CH prevalence [12,13]. Small for gestational age, especially, is a high risk for hyperthyrotropinemia [13]. The incidence of low birthweight was higher among infants with high TSH levels on NBS in our study than among the general population. However, all NBS-positive low-birthweight infants were able to discontinue LT4 replacement by the age of 15 years. Because high TSH levels in low-birthweight infants may be transient, these patients should be excluded when determining the prevalence of permanent CH.

Although this was not a nationwide survey, this is the first study to clarify the true prevalence of permanent CH in Japan. The study was limited by the inability to ascertain the LT4 replacement status in patients transferred to other hospitals, and the lack of investigation of the presence of CH patients who were not detected by NBS. We also did not examine factors associated with transient CH in this study. However, this study was strengthened by uniform data, as a single institution managed almost all the CH screenings in the Niigata Prefecture, and transient CH was excluded from long-term follow-up until the age of 15 years.

5. Conclusions

In our study, 62.5% of the LT4 replacement patients discontinued treatment by 15 years of age. From these results, the prevalence of permanent CH in the Niigata Prefecture during this period was 1 in 2500–3500 children.

Author Contributions: Conceptualization, K.N.; methodology, K.N., T.A., H.S., H.N., S.S., N.S., S.H. and K.S.; data curation, K.N.; writing—original draft preparation, K.N.; writing—review and editing, T.A., H.S., H.N., S.S., N.S., S.H. and K.S. All authors have read and agreed to the published version of the manuscript.

Funding: This research received no external funding.

Institutional Review Board Statement: The study was conducted according to the guidelines of the Declaration of Helsinki and approved by the Institutional Ethics Committee of Niigata University (protocol code: 2020-0497; date of approval: 29 April 2021).

Informed Consent Statement: Informed consent was obtained from the patients in an opt-out method for the publication of this paper.

Data Availability Statement: The data presented are available upon request from the corresponding author. The data are not publicly available because of privacy restrictions.

Acknowledgments: We would like to thank Keiko Hokari and Naoko Otabe of the Niigata Health Service Center for providing us with data on NBS in the Niigata Prefecture. We would like to thank all the patients who participated in this study.

Conflicts of Interest: The authors declare no conflict of interest.

References

1. Minamitani, K.; Inomata, H. Neonatal screening for congenital hypothyroidism in Japan. *Pediatr. Endocrinol. Rev.* **2012**, *10* (Suppl. 1), 79–88. [PubMed]
2. Minamitani, K.; Sugihara, S.; Inomata, H.; Harada, S. Re-evaluation of neonatal screening system for congenital hypothyroidism in Japan. *Jpn. J. Neonatal Screen.* **2009**, *19*, 51–57. (In Japanese)
3. Ford, G.; LaFranchi, S.H. Screening for congenital hypothyroidism: A worldwide view of strategies. *Best Pract. Res. Clin. Endocrinol. Metab.* **2014**, *28*, 175–187. [CrossRef] [PubMed]
4. Barry, Y.; Bonaldi, C.; Goulet, V.; Coutant, R.; Léger, J.; Paty, A.C.; Delmas, D.; Cheillan, D.; Roussey, M. Increased incidence of congenital hypothyroidism in France from 1982 to 2012: A nationwide multicenter analysis. *Ann. Epidemiol.* **2016**, *26*, 100–105. [CrossRef] [PubMed]
5. McGrath, N.; Hawkes, C.P.; McDonnell, C.M.; Cody, D.; O'Connell, S.M.; Mayne, P.D.; Murphy, N.P. Incidence of Congenital Hypothyroidism Over 37 Years in Ireland. *Pediatrics* **2018**, *142*, e20181199. [CrossRef] [PubMed]
6. Miki, K.; Nose, O.; Miyai, K.; Yabuuchi, H.; Harada, T. Transient infantile hyperthyrotrophinaemia. *Arch. Dis. Child.* **1989**, *64*, 1177–1182. [CrossRef] [PubMed]
7. Nagasaki, K.; Asami, T.; Ogawa, Y.; Kikuchi, T.; Uchiyama, M. A study of the etiology of congenital hypothyroidism in the Niigata prefecture of Japan in patients born between 1989 and 2005 and evaluated at ages 5–19. *Thyroid* **2011**, *21*, 361–365. [CrossRef] [PubMed]
8. Rastogi, M.V.; LaFranchi, S.H. Congenital hypothyroidism. *Orphanet J. Rare Dis.* **2010**, *5*, 17. [CrossRef] [PubMed]
9. Gaudino, R.; Garel, C.; Czernichow, P.; Léger, J. Proportion of various types of thyroid disorders among newborns with congenital hypothyroidism and normally located gland: A regional cohort study. *Clin. Endocrinol.* **2005**, *62*, 444–448. [CrossRef]
10. Saba, C.; Guilmin-Crepon, S.; Zénaty, D.; Martinerie, L.; Paulsen, A.; Simon, D.; Storey, C.; Dos Santos, S.; Haignere, J.; Mohamed, D.; et al. Early Determinants of Thyroid Function Outcomes in Children with Congenital Hypothyroidism and a Normally Located Thyroid Gland: A Regional Cohort Study. *Thyroid* **2018**, *28*, 959–967. [CrossRef]
11. Rabbiosi, S.; Vigone, M.C.; Cortinovis, F.; Zamproni, I.; Fugazzola, L.; Persani, L.; Corbetta, C.; Chiumello, G.; Weber, G. Congenital hypothyroidism with eutopic thyroid gland: Analysis of clinical and biochemical features at diagnosis and after re-evaluation. *J. Clin. Endocrinol. Metab.* **2013**, *98*, 1395–1402. [CrossRef]
12. Mitchell, M.L.; Hsu, H.W.; Sahai, I. Massachusetts Pediatric Endocrine Work Group. The increased incidence of congenital hypothyroidism: Fact or fancy? *Clin. Endocrinol.* **2011**, *75*, 806–810. [CrossRef] [PubMed]
13. Grob, F.; Gutiérrez, M.; Leguizamón, L.; Fabres, J. Hyperthyrotropinemia is common in preterm infants who are born small for gestational age. *J. Pediatr. Endocrinol. Metab.* **2020**, *33*, 375–382. [CrossRef] [PubMed]

Review

Thirty-Year Lessons from the Newborn Screening for Congenital Adrenal Hyperplasia (CAH) in Japan

Atsumi Tsuji-Hosokawa [1,2] and Kenichi Kashimada [2,*]

1. Department of Systems BioMedicine, National Research Institute for Child Health and Development, Tokyo 157-8535, Japan; tsuji-a@ncchd.go.jp
2. Department of Pediatrics and Developmental Biology, Tokyo Medical and Dental University (TMDU), Tokyo 113-8510, Japan
* Correspondence: kkashimada.ped@tmd.ac.jp

Abstract: Congenital adrenal hyperplasia (CAH) is an inherited disorder caused by the absence or severely impaired activity of steroidogenic enzymes involved in cortisol biosynthesis. More than 90% of cases result from 21-hydroxylase deficiency (21OHD). To prevent life-threatening adrenal crisis and to help perform appropriate sex assignments for affected female patients, newborn screening (NBS) programs for the classical form of CAH have been introduced in numerous countries. In Japan, the NBS for CAH was introduced in 1989, following the screenings for phenylketonuria and congenital hypothyroidism. In this review, we aim to summarize the experience of the past 30 years of the NBS for CAH in Japan, composed of four parts, 1: screening system in Japan, 2: the clinical outcomes for the patients with CAH, 3: various factors that would impact the NBS system, including timeline, false positive, and LC-MS/MS, 4: Database composition and improvement of the screening program.

Keywords: congenital adrenal hyperplasia; 21-hydroxylase deficiency; newborn screening

1. Introduction

Congenital adrenal hyperplasia (CAH) is an inherited disorder caused by the loss or severely impaired activity of steroidogenic enzymes involved in cortisol biosynthesis (Figure 1A,B) [1,2]. More than 90 percent of cases result from 21-hydroxylase deficiency (21OHD) caused by mutations in *CYP21A2*. The prevalence of 21OHD is estimated to be 1:15,000–16,000 in the USA and Europe [3] and slightly lower in Japan (1:18,000) [4–6]. The clinical spectrum of the disease ranges from the most severe to mild forms, depending upon the degree of enzyme deficiency [2].

The disease is mainly classified into two forms: classical and nonclassical. The classical form is associated with two major problems: life-threatening adrenal crisis in both sexes and virilization of the external genitalia in 46,XX patients. The classical form is further subdivided into two subtypes, the severest, salt wasting (SW) form, and simple virilizing (SV) form. The SW form is associated with cortisol and aldosterone deficiencies, in which neonates are likely to develop life-threatening adrenal crises with severe hyponatremia and hyperkalemia. Virilization of the external genitalia in newborn females and precocious puberty due to overproduction of androgens by the adrenal cortex are the other major clinical manifestations of the SW and SV forms. However, the clinical phenotypes of the SW type and the SV forms may overlap, and attempts to differentiate them based on endocrinological evaluation without genetic analysis are sometimes inconclusive [2].

To prevent a life-threatening adrenal crisis and help perform appropriate sex assignments for affected female patients, newborn screening (NBS) programs for the classical form of CAH have been introduced in numerous countries [7]. In Japan, the NBS for CAH was introduced in 1989, following that for PKU and congenital hypothyroidism [4].

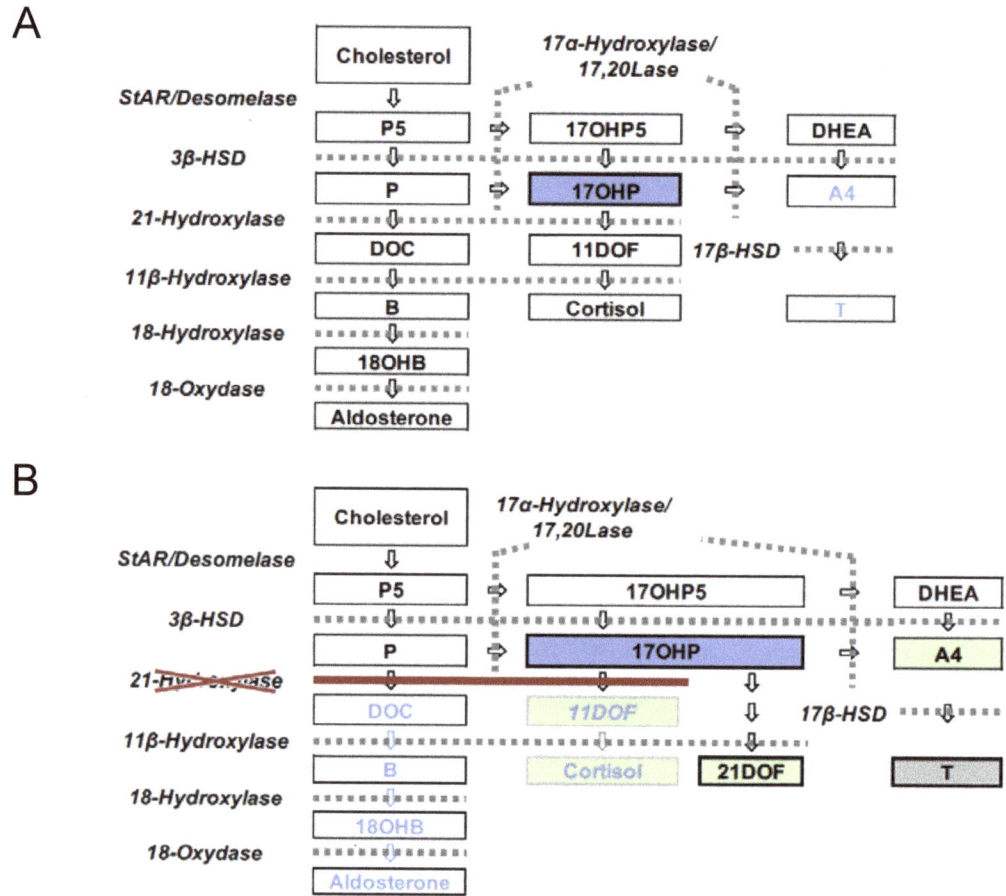

Figure 1. Steroid synthesis in the adrenal cortex (**A**) and the pathophysiology of 21OHD (**B**). P5: Pregnenolone, 17αOHP5: 17-hydroxypregnenolone, P: Progesterone, 17αOHP: 17-hydroxyprogesterone, DOC: Deoxycorticosterone, 11DOF: 11-deoxycortisol, B: Corticosterone, 18OHB: 18-Hydroxycorticosterone, DHEA: Dehydroepiandrostendione, A4: Androstenedione, T: Testosterone. 17αOHP and other green steroids are included in the panel of LC-MS/MS screening in Japan. Steroids written in blue suggest its synthesis is reduced.

In contrast to the classical form, the nonclassical form has a milder phenotype in which clinical problems are not obvious during the neonatal period or childhood, generally developing during adolescence or adulthood [1,2]. The prevalence of nonclassical form in Japan is estimated much lower than that in western countries [8–10]. Although some of them are screened by the NBS, the screening program is not designed to detect all the newborns with the nonclassical form.

The aim of this review is to summarize the experience of the past 30 years of the NBS for CAH in Japan, comprising four parts: 1, screening system in Japan; 2, clinical outcomes for patients with CAH; 3, factors that would impact the NBS system, including timeline, false positive, and LC-MS/MS; and 4, database composition and improvement of the screening program.

2. Screening System in Japan

The NBS in Japan was introduced individually into the prefectural administration according to a government notification by the Ministry of Health and Welfare in 1977. The basis of the NBS system, such as the timeline, and the screening panel are identical in all local governments. After informed consent is obtained from a legal guardian, blood samples are collected by a heel prick blotted on a filter paper from neonates at 4–7 days from birth, and the filter paper samples are immediately sent to a laboratory allocated by the prefectural government.

The details of the screening system are different among laboratories, and as a representative, the screening algorithm in Tokyo was shown in Figure 2. In Tokyo, the 1st screening is divided into two procedures. The level of 17-hydroxyprogesterone (17αOHP) is initially determined by enzyme-linked immunosorbent assay (ELISA) without steroid extraction. We select blood samples in the 97th percentile or higher for 17αOHP values for subjecting the second-tier test, which is carried out after steroid extraction [4,5,11,12]. The cutoff criteria for the second-tier test are shown in Table 1.

The NBS has two different cutoff values: for "screening positive" and for "retest". When the 17αOHP level is higher than the screening positive cutoff value, the neonate is directly referred to a pediatric endocrinologist for further endocrinological evaluation. Neonates with 17αOHP levels more than the retest cutoff value are retested. When the 17αOHP levels are higher than the retest cutoff value two–three times, the screening is considered positive (Figure 2) [4,5,11–13].

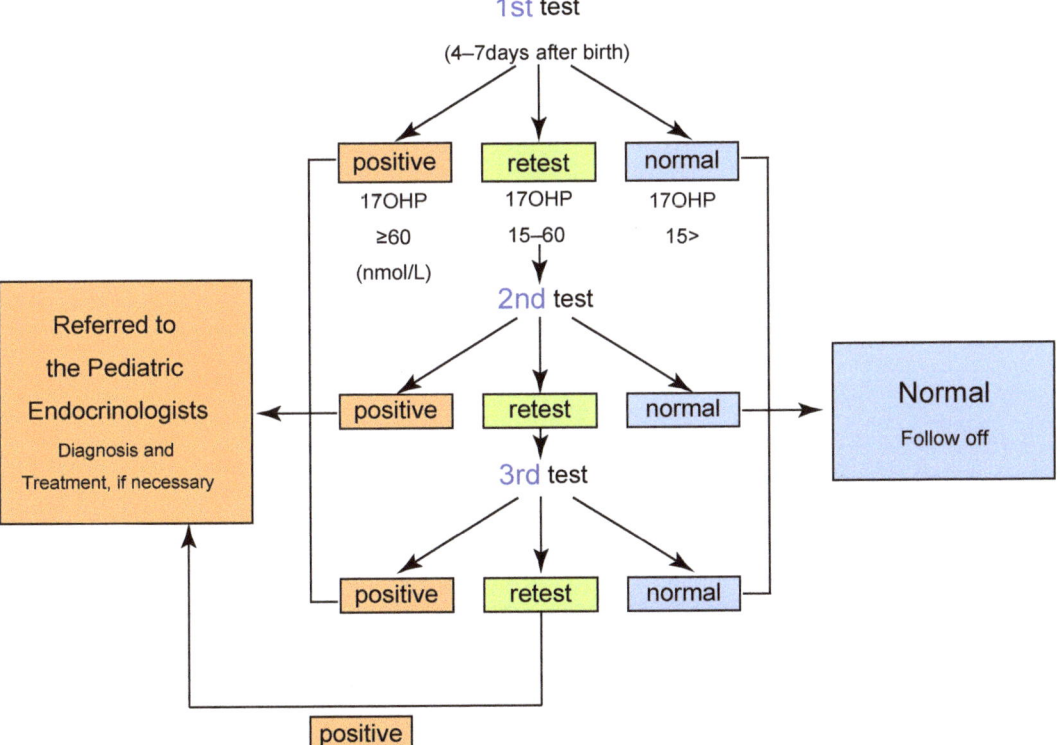

Figure 2. Algorithm of CAH screening in Tokyo.

In some female patients, blood sampling for the screening is performed ahead of schedule due to atypical genitalia, which is one of the major clinical symptoms in female neonates with 21OHD and is frequently recognized at birth.

To reduce the number of false-positive results in preterm newborns, one of the most serious issues in the screening for 21OHD, some laboratories, including that of Tokyo, employ cutoff values based on gestational age and/or birth weight. The cutoff values were determined according to a pilot study of serum 17αOHP levels in full-term and preterm infants. As a representative screening system in Japan, the algorithm and criteria for the screening in Tokyo are shown in Table 1 and Figure 2 [5], respectively.

Table 1. Criteria of CAH mass screening in Tokyo.

		<Criteria According to the Gestational Age>			
Gestational age at birth (weeks) [*1a]		≤29	30–34	35–36	≥37
Corrected gestational age (weeks) [*1b]		≤31	32–35	36–37	≥38
		<Criteria According to Weight> [*2,*3]			
Body weight (g)		≤999	1000–1999	2000–2499	≥2500
Cutoff level of 17αOHP [n·mol/L]	Retest [*4]	60	45	24	15
	Positive [*5]		60	60	60

[*1a] Samples collected before the age of 7 days, [*1b] Samples collected at the age of 7 days or after, [*2] 1st test: body weight = birth weight, 2nd test and after: body weight = corrected body weight calculated by the formula as below. Corrected body weight at test (g) = birth weight (g) + (age at test − 7) × 20 (g). [*3] For infants born small or large for gestational age, either the criteria of gestational age (corrected gestational age) or body weight was applied, whichever was a lower value. Since 2012, criteria according to weight have not been used, and solely gestational age-stratified cutoff has been used. [*4] recall for the second (or the third) test of the screening. [*5] refer to hospitals for further endocrinological examinations.

For the quality control of the screening, most screening laboratories perform follow-up surveys of the patients who were referred to hospitals. In the surveys, clinical information of the patients, including confirmed diagnosis, is collected from the pediatric endocrinologists at the hospitals [13].

3. Clinical Outcomes of the Newborn Screening for CAH in Japan

3.1. The Effects of the Screening

The clinical profiles of 21OHD before the introduction of the screening differ remarkably from the current profiles [14]. Before the introduction of the screening, Suwa S et al. conducted a nationwide survey and reported the clinical profiles of 21OHD in Japan. According to the survey, the estimated prevalence of 21OHD was 1/43,764, and the average age in days when the patients firstly visited the hospitals was 1102. In the SW type, the average age of the first hospital visit was 55 days (male: 63 days (range, 1 days to 3 years), female: 47 days (range: 0 days to 3.9 years)), and in the SV form, the average age at first visit was 6.4 years (male: 5.9 years (range: 14 days to 34 years), female: 6.5 years (range: 0 days to 44 years)) (Table 2) [15]. The ratio of male to female was 1:1.5, and the number of male patients was significantly lower than that of females, implying that a substantial number of male patients were missed, i.e., the SV form remained undiagnosed or the fatal cases with the SW form in the neonatal-infantile period. Consistently, the survey revealed that the mortality rate was 10.6% in neonates with the SW form, which is consistent with the reports from other countries [15]. In 46,XX cases, 12.9% were firstly assigned as male because of atypical genitalia and corrected to female sex after the diagnosis of 21OHD [15].

Table 2. Age at diagnosis before and after implementation of the screening.

	Before CAH Screening *			After CAH Screening **		
	Male	Female	Total	Male	Female	Total
SW type	63 days (120)	47 days (96)	55 days (216)	9.0 days (55)	6.2 days (45)	7.6 days (100)
SV type	5.0 yrs (39)	6.5 yrs (150)	6.4 yrs (189)			

Numbers in parentheses indicate numbers of the subjects, *, **: according to the data reported by Suwa et al., 1994 [15] and Gau et al., 2020 [13], respectively.

After the introduction of the screening, the clinical outcomes of 21OHD during the neonatal/infantile period were remarkably improved. The average ages at the first visit were 8.2 and 7.6 days (male: 9.2 days, female: 6.0 days) in Sapporo and Tokyo, respectively (Table 2) [6,13]. To date, no fatal cases have been identified.

Although the follow-up surveys and the screening systems are not designed for detecting false-negative cases, based on a survey for the literature and the annual reports from NBS programs, no false-negative cases have been reported since the introduction of the screening [5,6,13]. We presume that the sex of all 46,XX cases was correctly assigned.

3.2. The Progression of Salt Wasting during the First Two Weeks of Life

Adrenal crisis is a life-threatening medical emergency, and eradicating the lethal cases of 21OHD is one of the major goals of newborn screening [16]. Although the fact that there were no reported fatal cases suggests the primary goal of the screening has been accomplished, 37.4% of 21OHD neonates already developed severe salt wasting, which is defined by Na < 130 mEq/L, K > 7 mEq/L, on arrival at medical hospitals in Tokyo screening [13]. Furthermore, some of the 21OHD neonates exhibited life-threatening salt wasting, such as more than 10 mEq/L of serum K [13].

Severe adrenal crisis during the neonatal to early infantile period would cause neurological comorbidities. According to the nationwide survey before the introduction of NBS in Japan, a substantial number of the 21OHD patients revealed to have neurological comorbidities including intellectual disability and epilepsy. The prevalence associated with the SW form was higher, 18.5%, than with the SV form, 9.4%, suggesting that delayed diagnosis of adrenal crisis causes intellectual disability [17]. Consistently, in the retrospective study from the U.K., where NBS for 21OHD is not introduced, more than 20% of the SW-type 21OHD patients developed learning difficulties [14]. Those suggest that just eradication of lethal cases would not be sufficient for the goal of the 21OHD screening, and avoiding severe adrenal crisis should be considered.

Retrospective analysis of the follow-up survey of the NBS in Tokyo revealed that, in classical 21OHD patients, the serum Na and K levels linearly deteriorated with age in days, and the age when the regression lines reached Na < 130 mEq/L, K > 7 mEq/L approximately coincided at 11.1 and 12.3 days, respectively [13] (Figure 3). The risk of developing severe salt wasting increases during the second week of life without a threshold, and, therefore, an early intervention, ideally during the first week of life, is desirable [13,18,19].

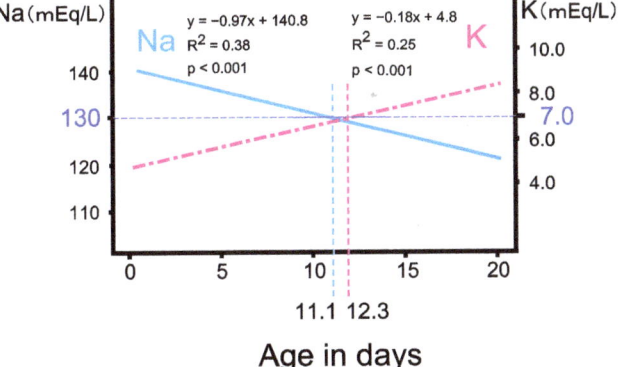

Figure 3. Clinical features of serum sodium (Na) and potassium (K) levels in 21OHD neonates. Retrospective analysis of the NBS in Tokyo revealed that, in classical 21OHD patients, the serum Na and K levels linearly deteriorated with age in days, and the age when the regression lines reached Na < 130 mEq/L, K > 7 mEq/L approximately coincided at 11.1 and 12.3 days, respectively. (Modified from Gau et al., 2020 [13]).

3.3. Triage of the Neonates with Salt Wasting by Body Weight Change

The follow-up survey in Tokyo revealed that from the second week of life, changes in body weight provide a useful index in the evaluation of neonates with positive CAH screening results [13]. Neonates with decreasing body weight from the birth weight are likely to have classical 21OHD, and neonates with increasing body weight after birth are more likely to be false positives [13]. Furthermore, even in cases of 21OHD, the possibility of developing severe salt wasting, such as hyponatremia (<130 mEq/L) or hyperkalemia (>7 mEq/L), is extremely low without loss of body weight (Figure 4). Contrary to body weight change, the relevance of predicting severe salt wasting based on the 17αOHP level is extremely low because the 17αOHP level is not associated with Na or K levels [13].

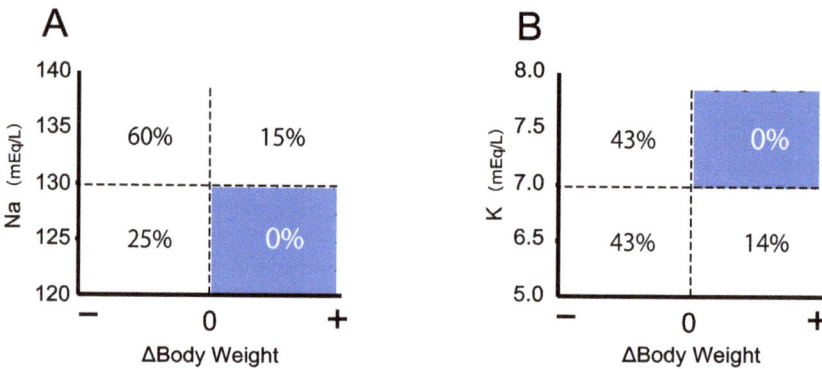

Figure 4. Body weight change from birth is an excellent predictor of 21OHD and the risk of severe salt wasting. Body weight data of 21OHD patients at 7–14 days after birth were collected, and the change in body weight from birth weight was examined. None of the 21OHD patients with severe salt wasting (Na < 130 meq/L or K > 7.0 mEq/L) exhibited increased body weight (**A**,**B**).

Although the findings of body weight change in patients cannot be the direct criteria for the CAH screening protocol, they may assist in some individual cases, e.g., for triaging a neonate with a positive result who is living in a region with limited access to a pediatric endocrinologist or in which there is no CAH screening.

4. Potential Issues of Testing Practices in the Newborn Screening for CAH in Japan

4.1. The Timeline of the Newborn Screening for 21OHD

The timeline of the NBSs is becoming earlier worldwide because newly added inborn errors to the screening panel require early intervention immediately after birth. In the U.S., SIMD (Society for Inherited Metabolic Disorders) defines the critical condition as a condition in which serious symptoms may present acutely in the first weeks of life with a short pre-symptomatic window and require immediate treatment to mitigate morbidity and mortality [20]. More than 10 inborn errors of organic acid disorders and fatty acid oxidation disorders are involved in the list, and the SIMD recommends considering the list as an important starting point for discussion between clinicians and laboratories [20]. Accordingly, blood samples for screening are collected 48 h after birth in the U.S., and the recommended age in days when the first results are obtained should be seven [21]. Indeed, in 2018, 64% of the first results were available within 5 days after birth (Table 3) [22]. The situation is similar in the EU, and, in most countries, blood sampling starts 72 h after birth (Table 3) [23].

In the NBS for 21OHD, several factors should be considered in terms of timing for the blood sampling. Especially, given the rate of 37.4% neonates with severe salt wasting in Japan, earlier sampling can be discussed for the prevention of life-threatening salt wasting. However, an increase in serum 17αOHP level has been observed in unaffected neonates during the first 1–2 days of life, and there is evidence of false negatives associated with the early collection of specimens in the U.S. [24]. Further, the timeline is determined by various factors of other diseases in the screening panels, which are different among countries (Table 3). For optimizing the timeline of the screening, we need careful discussion continuously.

Table 3. Summary of newborn screening in European countries, Oceania, and the U.S. (modified table from reference [25]) and the following website (https://www.hrsa.gov/advisory-committees/heritable-disorders/newborn-screening-timeliness.html, https://newbornscreening.hrsa.gov/your-state#w, https://www.newsteps.org/resources/data-visualizations/newborn-screening-status-all-disorders, visited date, "23 April 2021").

Countries [*1]	Approximate Population (Million)	Screening Panel					Interval Birth-Sampling				Interval Sampling Analysis					
		CAH	CH	PKU	GAL	AAD, OA, FAOD	<48 h	48–72 h	72–96 h	>96 h	1 d	2 d	3 d	4 d	5 d	>6 d
Austria	8.8	x [*2]	x	x	x	>6	x	x			x	x	x			
Belgium	10.5	x	x	x	x	>6		x	x	x	x					
Denmark	5.6	x	x	x	x	>6	x				x	x				
France	67	x	x	x	x	P [*2]		x			x	x				
Germany	80	x	x	x	x	>6	x	x			x	x				
Netherlands	17.8	x	x	x	x	>6			x		x	x	x			
Spain	46.5	x	x	x	P	>6	x	x	x			x	x	x	x	
Sweden	10	x	x	x	x	>6		x			x	x	x			
Switzerland	8.1	x	x	x	x	1–6			x		x					
Finland	5.5		x	x		>6	x [*4]	x	x	x	x	x	x	x		
Greece	10.5		x	x	x			x								x
Hungary	10		x	x	x	>6	x					x	x			
Ireland	4.9		x	x	x			x	x	x	x					
Italy	60.5		x	x	P	P		x			x	x	x	x		
Norway	5.3		x	x		>6	x					x				
Portugal	10.3		x	x		>6	x			x	x	x				
U.K.	66.6		x	x		1–6			x			x	x			
U.S. [*3]	328.2	50/50	50/50	50/50	50/50	50/50	x				x	x				
JPN	126.3	x	x	x	x	>6			x		x	x	x	x		

[*1] European countries whose population is approximately more than 5 million were listed. [*2] x (in screening panel section) = in screening panel, P = pilot/regional screening. [*3] In the United States section, the number of states that include the disease in the screening panel is listed. In the AAD, OA, and FAOD section, states that implemented more than six of the metabolic disorders were counted. The interval between birth, sampling, and analysis of U.S. is recommended timeline. [*4] Cord blood is used for some of the screening.

4.2. High Rate of False Positive

For the 17αOHP measurement, immunoassays have been used because of their sensitivity, cost, and simplicity. However, immunoassays lead to high rates of false positives, seriously affecting the screening efficiency [5,18,26].

One of the major reasons is the cross-reactivity with steroids, such as 17-hydroxy pregnenolone sulfate and 15β-hydroxylated compounds, which is high in preterm infants, and the ratio of false positives is extremely high in preterm infants. To minimize false positives, cutoff points stratified by gestational age and/or birth weight have been used in some screening systems. Although the stratified cutoff improves positive predictive value (PPV) to some extent, its efficiency is limited [5,27–30]. In the Tokyo system, gestational age and birth weight cutoff points have been used since the introduction of the NBS (Table 1). While the average PPV in Japan was reported as 6.6%, the Tokyo screening program achieved 25.8% (Figure 5). On the other hand, the PPV in preterm infants with a gestational age of ≤37 weeks was only 2% [5].

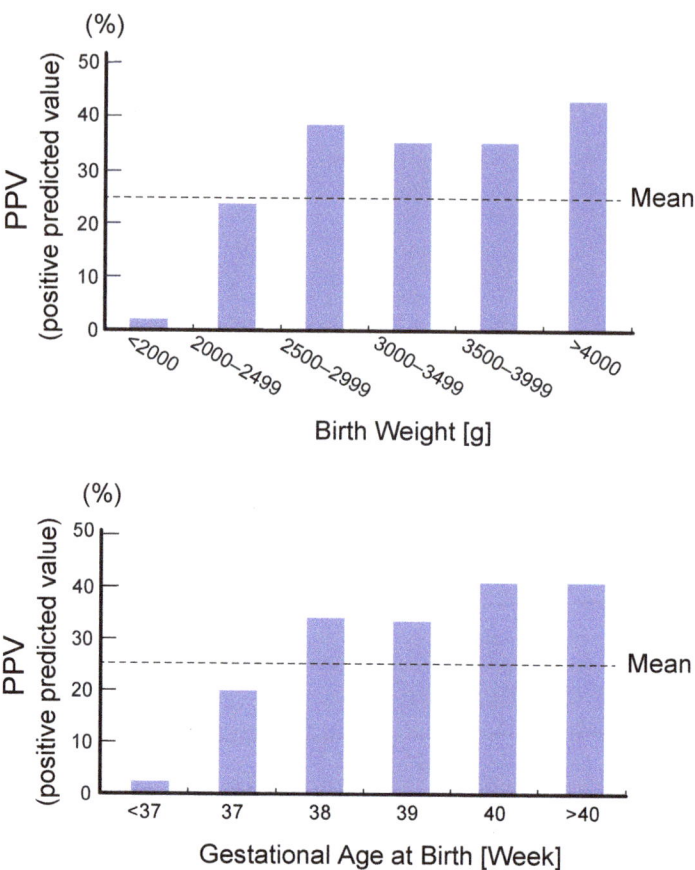

Figure 5. PPV (positive predicted value) of CAH screening in Tokyo according to the birth weights and the gestational ages of newborns judged as positive. (Modified from Tsuji et al., 2015 [5]).

Another cause for the high false-positive rate is the nature of 17αOHP itself. Historically, 17αOHP was originally considered as the pathogenic androgen in cases of 21OHD rather than as a diagnostic marker, and it has several shortcomings as a diagnostic for 21OHD [31]. The level of 17αOHP is high in cord blood during the first 1–2 days of life, and stress from other illnesses may result in the 17αOHP remaining high in unaffected neonates. Furthermore, in other forms of CAH, including 11-hydroxylase deficiency (11OHD), 3β-hydroxysteroid dehydrogenase deficiency (3βHSDD), and P450 oxidoreductase deficiency (PORD), 17αOHP may be elevated to almost the same level as that of 21OHD [32]. For further improving PPV in 21OHD screening, measuring other biomarkers with high specificity for 21OHD would be required.

4.3. LC-MS/MS Analysis of 17αOHP as a Second-Tier Test and Diagnostic Test for 21OHD

To improve PPV, an alternative methodology should measure disease-specific markers other than 17αOHP or has high specificity for the target steroids. When used appropriately under highly regulated conditions, liquid chromatography-tandem mass spectrometry (LC-MS/MS) is considered as the gold standard for steroids assays [33–39], and the guideline of the Endocrine Society have recommended to employ LC-MS/MS for measuring 17αOHP of the second tier in neonatal screening since 2018 [16].

In addition to its specificity, the advantage of LC-MS/MS is the capability for the simultaneous assay of multiple steroids [33,34,36]. In Japan, a steroid profile panel from

Siemens Healthineers AG (Frankfurt, Germany), "MS^2-screening CAH" was developed for the CAH screening. Five steroids were selected for the panel: 17αOHP, 21-deoxycortisol (21-DOF), 11-deoxycortisol (11-DOF), 4-androstenedione (4AD), and cortisol (F). Accordingly, the cutoff criteria of the LC-MS/MS assay are not solely based on 17αOHP, but on 21DOF and the ratios of steroids, such as (17αOHP + 4AD)/F, 11DOF/17αOHP (Table 4) [33]. The combination of highly specific LC-MS/MS and simultaneous assays of five steroids is expected to dramatically improve the efficiency of the screening [33,34,36].

Table 4. Cutoff level of 17αOHP and other steroids assayed by LC-MS/MS in Saitama, Sapporo and Tokyo, Japan *[1].

		Screening Positive Cutoff Level			
				Tokyo	
Prefecture		Saitama	Sapporo	Criteria A *[2,3]	Criteria B *[2,3]
17αOHP (ng/mL)	Term birth	>20	>20	>5	>5
	Preterm birth	>30	>50		
21DOF (ng/mL)		>1.0	>2.0	>1.0	
(17αOHP + 4AD)/F					>2.0
11DOF/17αOHP					<0.1
Retest Cutoff Level					
Prefecture			Saitama *[2]	Sapporo *[2]	Tokyo *[2]
17αOHP (ng/mL)			>1.0	>2.5	>1.5
(17αOHP + 4AD)/F			>0.1	>0.1	>0.3
11DOF/17αOHP			<0.3	<0.2	<0.3

*[1] The algorithm of the screening is the same as shown in Figure 1. When the retest values are documented twice, the patients are judged as positive. *[2] The result is judged as positive or retest when all parameters meet the criteria. *[3] The patient with the result that meets criteria A or B is considered as screening positive.

Indeed, the outcomes of LC-MS/MS are excellent. In 2018, the LC-MS/MS assay for 21OHD was employed in 5 of 37 prefectural laboratories in Japan. In immunoassay screening, out of 653 subjects with positive results, there were 38 confirmed cases of 21OHD, resulting in a PPV of 5.8% (38/653). On the other hand, the PPV in LC-MS/MS screening was 40.0% (6/15), indicating that the specificity of LC-MS/MS is remarkable [40]. Accordingly, in 2018, the Ministry of Health, Labor, and Welfare in Japan added LC-MS/MS to the list of recommended methodologies for the second-tier test of 21OHD screening [41].

In addition to improving the efficiency of 21OHD screening, the steroid profile assay by LC-MS/MS may bring further advantage to the screening, that is, assisting definitive diagnosis of 21OHD [34]. Although 21OHD can be diagnosed endocrinologically, the procedures and cutoff criteria are complicated because other rare forms of CAH, such as 11OHD, PORD, and 3βHSDD, should be differentiated from the diagnosis of 21OHD as we described in the previous section [32,42–48]. The nonspecific increase in 17αOHP levels in other forms of CAH has been considered as a potential clinical pitfall.

Currently, reliable methods for differentiating 21OHD from other forms of CAH are an adrenocorticotropic hormone (ACTH) stimulation test [16], urine steroid profile analyses using gas chromatography mass spectrometry [49], and genetic test, which cannot be used as a first-line diagnostic test because the procedure of *CYP21A2* gene analysis is extremely complicated [50–52].

It has been suggested that the ratios of steroids (17αOHP + 4AD)/F, 11-DOF/17αOHP, and 21-DOF may be more specific biomarkers for the diagnosis of 21OHD than that of 17αOHP and are expected to differentiate 21OHD from other types of CAH in which 17αOHP levels are elevated, such as 3βHSDD, 11OHD, and PORD. Although there are few reports of the levels of (17αOHP + 4AD)/F, 11-DOF/17αOHP, or 21-DOF in these forms of CAH, some cases suggest the potential usefulness of the five steroids in the screening panel. 21DOF would not be elevated in 3βHSDD because, in a model of partial 3βHSD deficiency preterm infants, 21DOF is not grossly elevated [34]. In patients with 11-OHD,

21-DOF levels are reported to be normal, and 11-DOF is markedly elevated, presumably increasing the 11-DOF/17αOHP ratio [53]. Urinary steroid profile analyses of PORD suggested that the ratio of pregnanetriolone (Ptl)/tetrahydrocortisone steroids (THEs) and a specific cutoff of 11β-hydroxyandrosterone (11HA) would be useful for differentiating PORD from 21OHD. Ptl, THEs, and 11HA are metabolites of 21DOF, 11DOF + cortisol, and 4AD, respectively, which are included in the LC-MS/MS screening panel [54].

Accordingly, in combination with other clinical symptoms and signs, such as poor body weight gain and high ACTH, 21OHD can be diagnosed based on the results of NBS by LC-MS/MS [31,34]. However, we cannot directly apply the screening criteria to the diagnostic criteria, and for establishing the diagnostic criteria, an accumulation of the cases is required.

5. Database Composition and Improvement of Screening Program

For better and more efficient management of the CAH, the screening programs need persistent improvement in quality. By examining reliable follow-up studies, the outcomes and the experiences of the screening should be retrospectively evaluated and shared among the screening laboratories [25,55,56]. For short-term outcomes, most laboratories and local governments have introduced follow-up surveys in Japan, using the results for more efficient screening by decreasing false positives and early availability of screening results.

On the other hand, the assessment of long-term outcomes for CAH patients identified by screening is challenging. A nationwide registry system is required to establish efficient long-term follow-up systems. In Japan, the current screening system depends on each local government; thus, the demanding task of organizing a cross-regional collaborative system that involves local governments, local laboratories, and medical institutes is required.

Recent studies have revealed that 21OHD patients have substantial risks for metabolic syndrome in adulthood [57–60]. The metabolic syndrome in 21OHD has been assumed to be due to long-term glucocorticoid therapy [61]. However, other causes, such as fetal environments, have also been suggested [62,63], and the pathophysiology of the condition remains unknown. Further, the quality of life of 21OHD patients in adulthood is largely unknown. Especially in female patients, their gender issues should be clarified in detail [64–66]. As mentioned previously, before the introduction of the screening, 21OHD patients had substantial risks for neurological sequelae, which are presumably caused by the adrenal crisis during the neonatal period [14,17]. Therefore, the introduction of NBS would reduce the risk for neurological sequelae [67], but currently, available data is limited. We should keep in mind that, even after the introduction of the screening, there are a substantial number of 21OHD patients who developed severe salt wasting before the introduction of therapy. Further, a recent study suggested the number of hyponatremic episodes is an independent risk for lower IQ, suggesting that for optimizing the management of 21OHD patients during childhood, preventing episodes of severe adrenal crisis is crucial [68]. Thus, clarifying long-term outcomes will provide valuable information for improving the screening logistics.

Long-term outcomes will also provide valuable insights for evaluating the cost-effectiveness of screening. Although several analyses have been performed economically, they were based on short-term outcomes with various analytical models, leading to inconsistent results [69–71]. In Japan, economic analyses based on detailed clinical data have not been performed. To better understand the cost-effectiveness of screening, comprehensive approaches based on long-term outcomes are essential.

Despite not covering 21OHD patients, the introduction of several registry systems for rare congenital diseases has encouraged us. In the EU, some international collaboration-based registry systems for rare congenital diseases, such as the European Registry and Network for Intoxication type Metabolic Diseases (E-IMD) and the European Registry and Network for Homocystinurias and Methylation Defects (E-HOD), have been established [25,72–75]. Further, the Japanese Society for Inherited Metabolic Disease has successfully introduced the registry system, "JaSMIn", for patients with inherited metabolic disease (https://www.jasmin-mcbank.com/, visited 23 April 2021). The limitation of this registry system is the unknown coverage rate due to voluntary patient registration. However, the registry is designed to cover a broad spectrum of rare inherited metabolic diseases that can be discovered by NBS, and it will provide valuable insights, enabling feedback on newborn screening in the future, including economic aspects.

Ideally, for establishing feedback systems with long-term follow-up surveys, close collaboration among the screening laboratory professionals, pediatricians, primary care providers, and clinical epidemiologists is essential [55,56,76,77]. Currently, to share the outcomes of the screening and updating of technical information, the Japan Society for Neonatal Screening has a collaborative laboratory integrated committee (Gijutsubu-kai). We expect that with this committee, pediatric endocrinologists and local governments would be able to construct large collaboration-based reports and infrastructure. A nationwide registry system in which all results of infants are registered and evaluated periodically would lead to further methodological improvements.

Author Contributions: Conceptualization, writing—original draft preparation, A.T.-H. and K.K.; supervision, K.K. Both authors have read and agreed to the published version of the manuscript.

Funding: The present study was partly supported by the grant from the Ministry of Health, Labour and Welfare of Japan (grant Nanbyo-Ippan046 to K.K. for research on intractable diseases, Principal Investigator: Tomonobu Hasegawa) (# 201811056A).

Data Availability Statement: The data presented in this study are available on request from the corresponding author. The data are not publicly available due to privacy policy.

Acknowledgments: We thank Masaru Fukushi for critical reading and valuable suggestions. We also thank Maki Gau (Tokyo Medical and Dental University), Nobuyuki Ishige (Tokyo Health Service Association, Newborn Screening), and Kazuhiro Watanabe (Tokyo Health Service Association, Newborn Screening) for valuable suggestions. We express our deep gratitude to the medical staff who provided the clinical information in the follow-up survey in Tokyo.

Conflicts of Interest: Atsumi Tsuji-Hosokawa received a research grant from the Japanese Society for Pediatric Endocrinology and Novo Nordisk Pharma Ltd. Kenichi Kashimada declare no conflict of interest.

Abbreviations

17αOHP	17-Hydroxyprogesterone
yrs	Years
CAH	Congenital adrenal hyperplasia
CH	Congenital hypothyroidism
PKU	Phenylketonuria
GAL	Galactosemia
AAD	Disorders of amino acid metabolism
OA	Disorders of organic acid metabolism
FAOD	Disorders of fatty acid metabolism

References

1. Speiser, P.W.; White, P.C. Congenital adrenal hyperplasia. *N. Engl. J. Med.* **2003**, *349*, 776–788. [CrossRef]
2. White, P.C.; Speiser, P.W. Congenital adrenal hyperplasia due to 21-hydroxylase deficiency. *Endocr. Rev.* **2000**, *21*, 245–291. [CrossRef] [PubMed]
3. van der Kamp, H.J.; Wit, J.M. Neonatal screening for congenital adrenal hyperplasia. *Eur. J. Endocrinol.* **2004**, *151* (Suppl. S3), U71–U75. [CrossRef]
4. Suwa, S. Nationwide survey of neonatal mass-screening for congenital adrenal hyperplasia in Japan. *Screening* **1994**, *3*, 141–151. [CrossRef]
5. Tsuji, A.; Konishi, K.; Hasegawa, S.; Anazawa, A.; Onishi, T.; Ono, M.; Morio, T.; Kitagawa, T.; Kashimada, K. Newborn screening for congenital adrenal hyperplasia in Tokyo, Japan from 1989 to 2013: A retrospective population-based study. *BMC Pediatr.* **2015**, *15*, 209. [CrossRef]

6. Morikawa, S.; Nakamura, A.; Fujikura, K.; Fukushi, M.; Hotsubo, T.; Miyata, J.; Ishizu, K.; Tajima, T. Results from 28 years of newborn screening for congenital adrenal hyperplasia in sapporo. *Clin. Pediatr. Endocrinol.* **2014**, *23*, 35–43. [CrossRef]
7. Clayton, P.E.; Miller, W.L.; Oberfield, S.E.; Ritzen, E.M.; Sippell, W.G.; Speiser, P.W.; Group, E.L.C.W. Consensus statement on 21-hydroxylase deficiency from the European Society for Paediatric Endocrinology and the Lawson Wilkins Pediatric Endocrine Society. *Horm. Res.* **2002**, *58*, 188–195. [CrossRef] [PubMed]
8. Tajima, T.; Fujieda, K.; Nakae, J.; Mikami, A.; Cutler, G.B., Jr. Mutations of the CYP21 gene in nonclassical steroid 21-hydroxylase deficiency in Japan. *Endocr. J.* **1998**, *45*, 493–497. [CrossRef] [PubMed]
9. Tajima, T.; Fujieda, K.; Nakae, J.; Toyoura, T.; Shimozawa, K.; Kusuda, S.; Goji, K.; Nagashima, T.; Cutler, G.B., Jr. Molecular basis of nonclassical steroid 21-hydroxylase deficiency detected by neonatal mass screening in Japan. *J. Clin. Endocrinol. Metab.* **1997**, *82*, 2350–2356. [CrossRef]
10. Kashimada, K.; Ishii, T.; Nagasaki, K.; Ono, M.; Tajima, T.; Yokota, I.; Hasegawa, Y. Clinical, biochemical, and genetic features of non-classical 21-hydroxylase deficiency in Japanese children. *Endocr. J.* **2015**, *62*, 277–282. [CrossRef]
11. Tajima, T.; Fujikura, K.; Fukushi, M.; Hotsubo, T.; Mitsuhashi, Y. Neonatal screening for congenital adrenal hyperplasia in Japan. *Pediatr. Endocrinol. Rev.* **2012**, *10* (Suppl. S1), 72–78. [PubMed]
12. Tajima, T.; Fukushi, M. Neonatal mass screening for 21-hydroxylase deficiency. *Clin. Pediatr. Endocrinol.* **2016**, *25*, 1–8. [CrossRef]
13. Gau, M.; Konishi, K.; Takasawa, K.; Nakagawa, R.; Tsuji-Hosokawa, A.; Hashimoto, A.; Sutani, A.; Tajima, T.; Hasegawa, T.; Morio, T.; et al. The progression of salt wasting and the body weight change during the first two weeks of life in classical 21-hydroxylase deficiency patients. *Clin. Endocrinol.* **2020**, *94*, 229–236. [CrossRef]
14. Donaldson, M.D.; Thomas, P.H.; Love, J.G.; Murray, G.D.; McNinch, A.W.; Savage, D.C. Presentation, acute illness, and learning difficulties in salt wasting 21-hydroxylase deficiency. *Arch. Dis. Child.* **1994**, *70*, 214–218. [CrossRef]
15. Suwa, S. Congenital adrenal hyperplasia. *Shouni Naika* **1994**, *26*, 1967–1972. (In Japanese)
16. Speiser, P.W.; Arlt, W.; Auchus, R.J.; Baskin, L.S.; Conway, G.S.; Merke, D.P.; Meyer-Bahlburg, H.F.L.; Miller, W.L.; Murad, M.H.; Oberfield, S.E.; et al. Congenital adrenal hyperplasia due to steroid 21-hydroxylase deficiency: An endocrine society clinical practice guideline. *J. Clin. Endocrinol. Metab.* **2018**, *103*, 4043–4088. [CrossRef]
17. Suwa, S.; Maesaka, H.; Suzuki, J.; Katsumata, N. A suvery report: The comrbidities of congenital adrenal hyperplasia. In *A Study for Newborn Screening, Annual Report in 1995*; The Japanese Ministry of Health, Labour and Welfare's Study Group for Physical and Mental Disabilities: Tokyo, Japan, 1985; pp. 274–277. (In Japanese)
18. Heather, N.L.; Seneviratne, S.N.; Webster, D.; Derraik, J.G.; Jefferies, C.; Carll, J.; Jiang, Y.; Cutfield, W.S.; Hofman, P.L. Newborn screening for congenital adrenal hyperplasia in New Zealand, 1994–2013. *J. Clin. Endocrinol. Metab.* **2015**, *100*, 1002–1008. [CrossRef]
19. Shima, R.; Sawano, K.; Shibata, N.; Nyuzuki, H.; Sasaki, S.; Sato, H.; Ogawa, Y.; Abe, Y.; Nagasaki, K.; Saitoh, A. Timing of hyponatremia development in patients with salt-wasting-type 21-hydroxylase deficiency. *Clin. Pediatr. Endocrinol.* **2020**, *29*, 105–110. [CrossRef] [PubMed]
20. Freedenberg, D.; Berry, S.; Dimmock, D.; Gibson, J.; Greene, C.; Kronn, D.; Tanksley, S. Society for Inherited Metabolic Disorders (SIMD) Position Statement, 2014: Identifying Abnormal Newborn Screens Requiring Immediate Notification of the Health Care Provider. Available online: https://www.simd.org/Issues/SIMD%20NBS%20Critical%20Conditions%20policy%20statement.pdf (accessed on 23 April 2021).
21. HRSA, F.A.C. Newborn Screening Timeliness Goals. Available online: https://www.hrsa.gov/advisory-committees/heritable-disorders/newborn-screening-timeliness.html (accessed on 20 May 2021).
22. Sontag, M.K.; Miller, J.I.; McKasson, S.; Sheller, R.; Edelman, S.; Yusuf, C.; Singh, S.; Sarkar, D.; Bocchini, J.; Scott, J.; et al. Newborn screening timeliness quality improvement initiative: Impact of national recommendations and data repository. *PLoS ONE* **2020**, *15*, e0231050. [CrossRef] [PubMed]
23. Loeber, J.G. Current Status of Newborn Screening in Europe (Based on an ISNS Survey Held during 2018). Available online: https://www.isns-neoscreening.org/wp-content/uploads/2019/04/NBS-in-Europe-2018.pdf (accessed on 5 October 2020).
24. Held, P.K.; Bird, I.M.; Heather, N.L. Newborn screening for congenital adrenal hyperplasia: Review of factors affecting screening accuracy. *Int. J. Neonatal. Screen* **2020**, *6*, 67. [CrossRef]
25. Loeber, J.G.; Platis, D.; Zetterstrom, R.H.; Almashanu, S.; Boemer, F.; Bonham, J.R.; Borde, P.; Brincat, I.; Cheillan, D.; Dekkers, E.; et al. Neonatal screening in Europe revisited: An ISNS perspective on the current state and developments since 2010. *Int. J. Neonatal. Screen* **2021**, *7*, 15. [CrossRef]
26. Coulm, B.; Coste, J.; Tardy, V.; Ecosse, E.; Roussey, M.; Morel, Y.; Carel, J.C.; Group, D.S. Efficiency of neonatal screening for congenital adrenal hyperplasia due to 21-hydroxylase deficiency in children born in mainland France between 1996 and 2003. *Arch. Pediatr. Adolesc. Med.* **2012**, *166*, 113–120. [CrossRef] [PubMed]
27. Pode-Shakked, N.; Blau, A.; Pode-Shakked, B.; Tiosano, D.; Weintrob, N.; Eyal, O.; Zung, A.; Levy-Khademi, F.; Tenenbaum-Rakover, Y.; Zangen, D.; et al. Combined gestational age- and birth weight-adjusted cutoffs for newborn screening of congenital adrenal hyperplasia. *J. Clin. Endocrinol. Metab.* **2019**, *104*, 3172–3180. [CrossRef]
28. van der Kamp, H.J.; Oudshoorn, C.G.; Elvers, B.H.; van Baarle, M.; Otten, B.J.; Wit, J.M.; Verkerk, P.H. Cutoff levels of 17-alpha-hydroxyprogesterone in neonatal screening for congenital adrenal hyperplasia should be based on gestational age rather than on birth weight. *J. Clin. Endocrinol. Metab.* **2005**, *90*, 3904–3907. [CrossRef]

29. Nordenstrom, A.; Wedell, A.; Hagenfeldt, L.; Marcus, C.; Larsson, A. Neonatal screening for congenital adrenal hyperplasia: 17-hydroxyprogesterone levels and CYP21 genotypes in preterm infants. *Pediatrics* **2001**, *108*, e68. [CrossRef]
30. Allen, D.B.; Hoffman, G.L.; Fitzpatrick, P.; Laessig, R.; Maby, S.; Slyper, A. Improved precision of newborn screening for congenital adrenal hyperplasia using weight-adjusted criteria for 17-hydroxyprogesterone levels. *J. Pediatr.* **1997**, *130*, 128–133. [CrossRef]
31. Miller, W.L. Congenital adrenal hyperplasia: Time to replace 17OHP with 21-deoxycortisol. *Horm. Res. Paediatr.* **2019**, *91*, 416–420. [CrossRef]
32. Takasawa, K.; Ono, M.; Hijikata, A.; Matsubara, Y.; Katsumata, N.; Takagi, M.; Morio, T.; Ohara, O.; Kashimada, K.; Mizutani, S. Two novel HSD3B2 missense mutations with diverse residual enzymatic activities for Delta5-steroids. *Clin. Endocrinol.* **2014**, *80*, 782–789. [CrossRef] [PubMed]
33. Higashi, T.; Nishio, T.; Uchida, S.; Shimada, K.; Fukushi, M.; Maeda, M. Simultaneous determination of 17alpha-hydroxypregnenolone and 17alpha-hydroxyprogesterone in dried blood spots from low birth weight infants using LC-MS/MS. *J. Pharm. Biomed. Anal.* **2008**, *48*, 177–182. [CrossRef]
34. Janzen, N.; Peter, M.; Sander, S.; Steuerwald, U.; Terhardt, M.; Holtkamp, U.; Sander, J. Newborn screening for congenital adrenal hyperplasia: Additional steroid profile using liquid chromatography-tandem mass spectrometry. *J. Clin. Endocrinol. Metab.* **2007**, *92*, 2581–2589. [CrossRef]
35. Kulle, A.E.; Riepe, F.G.; Hedderich, J.; Sippell, W.G.; Schmitz, J.; Niermeyer, L.; Holterhus, P.M. LC-MS/MS based determination of basal- and ACTH-stimulated plasma concentrations of 11 steroid hormones: Implications for detecting heterozygote CYP21A2 mutation carriers. *Eur. J. Endocrinol.* **2015**, *173*, 517–524. [CrossRef]
36. Monostori, P.; Szabo, P.; Marginean, O.; Bereczki, C.; Karg, E. Concurrent confirmation and differential diagnosis of congenital adrenal hyperplasia from dried blood spots: Application of a second-tier LC-MS/MS assay in a cross-border cooperation for newborn screening. *Horm. Res. Paediatr.* **2015**, *84*, 311–318. [CrossRef] [PubMed]
37. Lai, C.C.; Tsai, C.H.; Tsai, F.J.; Wu, J.Y.; Lin, W.D.; Lee, C.C. Rapid screening assay of congenital adrenal hyperplasia by measuring 17 alpha-hydroxyprogesterone with high-performance liquid chromatography/electrospray ionization tandem mass spectrometry from dried blood spots. *J. Clin. Lab. Anal.* **2002**, *16*, 20–25. [CrossRef]
38. Lacey, J.M.; Minutti, C.Z.; Magera, M.J.; Tauscher, A.L.; Casetta, B.; McCann, M.; Lymp, J.; Hahn, S.H.; Rinaldo, P.; Matern, D. Improved specificity of newborn screening for congenital adrenal hyperplasia by second-tier steroid profiling using tandem mass spectrometry. *Clin. Chem.* **2004**, *50*, 621–625. [CrossRef] [PubMed]
39. Minutti, C.Z.; Lacey, J.M.; Magera, M.J.; Hahn, S.H.; McCann, M.; Schulze, A.; Cheillan, D.; Dorche, C.; Chace, D.H.; Lymp, J.F.; et al. Steroid profiling by tandem mass spectrometry improves the positive predictive value of newborn screening for congenital adrenal hyperplasia. *J. Clin. Endocrinol. Metab.* **2004**, *89*, 3687–3693. [CrossRef] [PubMed]
40. Fukushi, M.; Isobe, M.; Kanda, K.; Saraie, H.; Fujikura, K.; Mitsui, N.; Mae, H.; Yamagami, Y. The quality control of LC-MS/MS screening for CAH as the second tier test. In Proceedings of the 47th Annual meeting of Japan Society for Neonatal Screening, Gifu, Japan, 25–26 September 2020.
41. Children and Families Bureau, Labour and Welfare in Japan. Notification for Newborn Screening, 2018. Notification from Director of the Maternal and Child Health Division. Available online: https://www.jsms.gr.jp/download/MHLW_MCH_20180330.pdf (accessed on 23 April 2021). (In Japanese)
42. Therrell, B.L., Jr.; Berenbaum, S.A.; Manter-Kapanke, V.; Simmank, J.; Korman, K.; Prentice, L.; Gonzalez, J.; Gunn, S. Results of screening 1.9 million Texas newborns for 21-hydroxylase-deficient congenital adrenal hyperplasia. *Pediatrics* **1998**, *101*, 583–590. [CrossRef] [PubMed]
43. Honour, J.W.; Anderson, J.M.; Shackleton, C.H. Difficulties in the diagnosis of congenital adrenal hyperplasia in early infancy: The 11 beta-hydroxylase defect. *Acta Endocrinol.* **1983**, *103*, 101–109. [CrossRef]
44. Tonetto-Fernandes, V.; Lemos-Marini, S.H.; Kuperman, H.; Ribeiro-Neto, L.M.; Verreschi, I.T.; Kater, C.E. Serum 21-Deoxycortisol, 17-Hydroxyprogesterone, and 11-deoxycortisol in classic congenital adrenal hyperplasia: Clinical and hormonal correlations and identification of patients with 11beta-hydroxylase deficiency among a large group with alleged 21-hydroxylase deficiency. *J. Clin. Endocrinol. Metab.* **2006**, *91*, 2179–2184. [CrossRef]
45. Homma, K.; Hasegawa, T.; Nagai, T.; Adachi, M.; Horikawa, R.; Fujiwara, I.; Tajima, T.; Takeda, R.; Fukami, M.; Ogata, T. Urine steroid hormone profile analysis in cytochrome P450 oxidoreductase deficiency: Implication for the backdoor pathway to dihydrotestosterone. *J. Clin. Endocrinol. Metab.* **2006**, *91*, 2643–2649. [CrossRef]
46. Fluck, C.E.; Tajima, T.; Pandey, A.V.; Arlt, W.; Okuhara, K.; Verge, C.F.; Jabs, E.W.; Mendonca, B.B.; Fujieda, K.; Miller, W.L. Mutant P450 oxidoreductase causes disordered steroidogenesis with and without Antley-Bixler syndrome. *Nat. Genet.* **2004**, *36*, 228–230. [CrossRef]
47. Jeandron, D.D.; Sahakitrungruang, T. A novel homozygous Q334X mutation in the HSD3B2 gene causing classic 3beta-hydroxysteroid dehydrogenase deficiency: An unexpected diagnosis after a positive newborn screen for 21-hydroxylase deficiency. *Horm. Res. Paediatr.* **2012**, *77*, 334–338. [CrossRef]
48. Cara, J.F.; Moshang, T., Jr.; Bongiovanni, A.M.; Marx, B.S. Elevated 17-hydroxyprogesterone and testosterone in a newborn with 3-beta-hydroxysteroid dehydrogenase deficiency. *N. Engl. J. Med.* **1985**, *313*, 618–621. [CrossRef]
49. Homma, K.; Hasegawa, T.; Takeshita, E.; Watanabe, K.; Anzo, M.; Toyoura, T.; Jinno, K.; Ohashi, T.; Hamajima, T.; Takahashi, Y.; et al. Elevated urine pregnanetriolone definitively establishes the diagnosis of classical 21-hydroxylase deficiency in term and preterm neonates. *J. Clin. Endocrinol. Metab.* **2004**, *89*, 6087–6091. [CrossRef]

50. Pignatelli, D.; Carvalho, B.L.; Palmeiro, A.; Barros, A.; Guerreiro, S.G.; Macut, D. The Complexities in Genotyping of Congenital Adrenal Hyperplasia: 21-Hydroxylase Deficiency. *Front. Endocrinol.* **2019**, *10*, 432. [CrossRef] [PubMed]
51. Parajes, S.; Quinterio, C.; Dominguez, F.; Loidi, L. A simple and robust quantitative PCR assay to determine CYP21A2 gene dose in the diagnosis of 21-hydroxylase deficiency. *Clin. Chem.* **2007**, *53*, 1577–1584. [CrossRef] [PubMed]
52. Gao, Y.; Lu, L.; Yu, B.; Mao, J.; Wang, X.; Nie, M.; Wu, X. The prevalence of the chimeric TNXA/TNXB gene and clinical symptoms of ehlers-danlos syndrome with 21-hydroxylase deficiency. *J. Clin. Endocrinol. Metab.* **2020**, *105*, 2288–2299. [CrossRef] [PubMed]
53. Janzen, N.; Riepe, F.G.; Peter, M.; Sander, S.; Steuerwald, U.; Korsch, E.; Krull, F.; Muller, H.L.; Heger, S.; Brack, C.; et al. Neonatal screening: Identification of children with 11beta-hydroxylase deficiency by second-tier testing. *Horm. Res. Paediatr.* **2012**, *77*, 195–199. [CrossRef]
54. Koyama, Y.; Homma, K.; Fukami, M.; Miwa, M.; Ikeda, K.; Ogata, T.; Hasegawa, T.; Murata, M. Two-step biochemical differential diagnosis of classic 21-hydroxylase deficiency and cytochrome P450 oxidoreductase deficiency in Japanese infants by GC-MS measurement of urinary pregnanetriolone/ tetrahydroxycortisone ratio and 11beta-hydroxyandrosterone. *Clin. Chem.* **2012**, *58*, 741–747. [CrossRef]
55. Burgard, P.; Rupp, K.; Lindner, M.; Haege, G.; Rigter, T.; Weinreich, S.S.; Loeber, J.G.; Taruscio, D.; Vittozzi, L.; Cornel, M.C.; et al. Newborn screening programmes in Europe; arguments and efforts regarding harmonization. Part 2. From screening laboratory results to treatment, follow-up and quality assurance. *J. Inherit. Metab. Dis.* **2012**, *35*, 613–625. [CrossRef] [PubMed]
56. Advisory Committee on Heritable Disorders in Newborns and Children; Zuckerman, A.E.; Badawi, D.; Brosco, J.P.; Brower, A.; Eichwald, J.; Feuchtbaum, L.; Finitzo, T.; Flannery, D.; Green, N.; et al. The Role of Quality Measures to Promote Long-Term Follow-up of Children Identified by Newborn Screening Programs; Advisory Committee on Heritable Disorders in Newborns and Children Advisory Committee on Heritable Disorders in Newborns and Children. 2018. Available online: https://www.hrsa.gov/sites/default/files/hrsa/advisory-committees/heritable-disorders/reports-recommendations/reports/role-of-quality-measures-in-nbs-sept2018-508c.pdf\T1\textquotedblright (accessed on 23 April 2021).
57. Stikkelbroeck, N.M.; Oyen, W.J.; van der Wilt, G.J.; Hermus, A.R.; Otten, B.J. Normal bone mineral density and lean body mass, but increased fat mass, in young adult patients with congenital adrenal hyperplasia. *J. Clin. Endocrinol. Metab.* **2003**, *88*, 1036–1042. [CrossRef]
58. Charmandari, E.; Chrousos, G.P. Metabolic syndrome manifestations in classic congenital adrenal hyperplasia: Do they predispose to atherosclerotic cardiovascular disease and secondary polycystic ovary syndrome? *Ann. N. Y. Acad. Sci.* **2006**, *1083*, 37–53. [CrossRef]
59. Zimmermann, A.; Grigorescu-Sido, P.; AlKhzouz, C.; Patberg, K.; Bucerzan, S.; Schulze, E.; Zimmermann, T.; Rossmann, H.; Geiss, H.C.; Lackner, K.J.; et al. Alterations in lipid and carbohydrate metabolism in patients with classic congenital adrenal hyperplasia due to 21-hydroxylase deficiency. *Horm. Res. Paediatr.* **2010**, *74*, 41–49. [CrossRef]
60. Finkielstain, G.P.; Kim, M.S.; Sinaii, N.; Nishitani, M.; Van Ryzin, C.; Hill, S.C.; Reynolds, J.C.; Hanna, R.M.; Merke, D.P. Clinical characteristics of a cohort of 244 patients with congenital adrenal hyperplasia. *J. Clin. Endocrinol. Metab.* **2012**, *97*, 4429–4438. [CrossRef] [PubMed]
61. Merke, D.P.; Bornstein, S.R. Congenital adrenal hyperplasia. *Lancet* **2005**, *365*, 2125–2136. [CrossRef]
62. Khalid, J.M.; Oerton, J.M.; Dezateux, C.; Hindmarsh, P.C.; Kelnar, C.J.; Knowles, R.L. Incidence and clinical features of congenital adrenal hyperplasia in Great Britain. *Arch. Dis. Child.* **2012**, *97*, 101–106. [CrossRef] [PubMed]
63. Takishima, S.; Nakajima, K.; Nomura, R.; Tsuji-Hosokawa, A.; Matsuda, N.; Matsubara, Y.; Ono, M.; Miyai, K.; Takasawa, K.; Morio, T.; et al. Lower body weight and BMI at birth were associated with early adiposity rebound in 21-hydroxylase deficiency patients. *Endocr. J.* **2016**, *63*, 983–990. [CrossRef] [PubMed]
64. Pasterski, V.; Zucker, K.J.; Hindmarsh, P.C.; Hughes, I.A.; Acerini, C.; Spencer, D.; Neufeld, S.; Hines, M. Increased cross-gender identification independent of gender role behavior in girls with congenital adrenal hyperplasia: Results from a standardized assessment of 4- to 11-year-old children. *Arch. Sex. Behav.* **2015**, *44*, 1363–1375. [CrossRef]
65. Meyer-Bahlburg, H.F.; Dolezal, C.; Baker, S.W.; Ehrhardt, A.A.; New, M.I. Gender development in women with congenital adrenal hyperplasia as a function of disorder severity. *Arch. Sex. Behav.* **2006**, *35*, 667–684. [CrossRef] [PubMed]
66. Meyer-Bahlburg, H.F.; Dolezal, C.; Baker, S.W.; New, M.I. Sexual orientation in women with classical or non-classical congenital adrenal hyperplasia as a function of degree of prenatal androgen excess. *Arch. Sex. Behav.* **2008**, *37*, 85–99. [CrossRef]
67. Harasymiw, L.A.; Grosse, S.D.; Sarafoglou, K. Attention-deficit/hyperactivity disorder among US children and adolescents with congenital adrenal hyperplasia. *J. Endocr. Soc.* **2020**, *4*, bvaa152. [CrossRef]
68. Hamed, S.A.; Metwalley, K.A.; Farghaly, H.S. Cognitive function in children with classic congenital adrenal hyperplasia. *Eur. J. Pediatr.* **2018**, *177*, 1633–1640. [CrossRef]
69. Fox, D.A.; Ronsley, R.; Khowaja, A.R.; Haim, A.; Vallance, H.; Sinclair, G.; Amed, S. Clinical impact and cost efficacy of newborn screening for congenital adrenal hyperplasia. *J. Pediatr.* **2020**, *220*, 101–108.e2. [CrossRef] [PubMed]
70. Carroll, A.E.; Downs, S.M. Comprehensive cost-utility analysis of newborn screening strategies. *Pediatrics* **2006**, *117*, S287–S295. [CrossRef] [PubMed]
71. Yoo, B.K.; Grosse, S.D. The cost effectiveness of screening newborns for congenital adrenal hyperplasia. *Public Health Genom.* **2009**, *12*, 67–72. [CrossRef] [PubMed]

72. Huemer, M.; Diodato, D.; Martinelli, D.; Olivieri, G.; Blom, H.; Gleich, F.; Kolker, S.; Kozich, V.; Morris, A.A.; Seifert, B.; et al. Phenotype, treatment practice and outcome in the cobalamin-dependent remethylation disorders and MTHFR deficiency: Data from the E-HOD registry. *J. Inherit. Metab. Dis.* **2019**, *42*, 333–352. [CrossRef]
73. Posset, R.; Garbade, S.F.; Gleich, F.; Gropman, A.L.; de Lonlay, P.; Hoffmann, G.F.; Garcia-Cazorla, A.; Nagamani, S.C.S.; Baumgartner, M.R.; Schulze, A.; et al. Long-term effects of medical management on growth and weight in individuals with urea cycle disorders. *Sci. Rep.* **2020**, *10*, 11948. [CrossRef]
74. Kolker, S.; Dobbelaere, D.; Haberle, J.; Burgard, P.; Gleich, F.; Summar, M.L.; Hannigan, S.; Parker, S.; Chakrapani, A.; Baumgartner, M.R.; et al. Networking across borders for individuals with organic acidurias and urea cycle disorders: The E-IMD consortium. *JIMD Rep.* **2015**, *22*, 29–38. [CrossRef] [PubMed]
75. Kozich, V.; Sokolova, J.; Morris, A.A.M.; Pavlikova, M.; Gleich, F.; Kolker, S.; Krijt, J.; Dionisi-Vici, C.; Baumgartner, M.R.; Blom, H.J.; et al. Cystathionine beta-synthase deficiency in the E-HOD registry-part I: Pyridoxine responsiveness as a determinant of biochemical and clinical phenotype at diagnosis. *J. Inherit. Metab. Dis.* **2021**, *44*, 677–692. [CrossRef]
76. Hoff, T.; Hoyt, A.; Therrell, B.; Ayoob, M. Exploring barriers to long-term follow-up in newborn screening programs. *Genet. Med.* **2006**, *8*, 563–570. [CrossRef]
77. Loeber, J.G.; Burgard, P.; Cornel, M.C.; Rigter, T.; Weinreich, S.S.; Rupp, K.; Hoffmann, G.F.; Vittozzi, L. Newborn screening programmes in Europe; arguments and efforts regarding harmonization. Part 1. From blood spot to screening result. *J. Inherit. Metab. Dis.* **2012**, *35*, 603–611. [CrossRef]

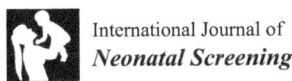

Article

Development of Second-Tier Liquid Chromatography-Tandem Mass Spectrometry Analysis for Expanded Newborn Screening in Japan

Yosuke Shigematsu [1,2,*], Miori Yuasa [1], Nobuyuki Ishige [3], Hideki Nakajima [4] and Go Tajima [4]

1. Department of Pediatrics, Faculty of Medical Sciences, University of Fukui, Fukui 910-1193, Japan; miori@u-fukui.ac.jp
2. Department of Pediatrics, Uji-Tokushukai Medical Center, Uji 611-0041, Japan
3. Division of Newborn Screening, Tokyo Health Service Association, Tokyo 162-8402, Japan; novi.burgi-1579@snow.email.ne.jp
4. Division of Neonatal Screening, Research Institute, National Center for Child Health and Development, Tokyo 157-8535, Japan; nakajima-h@ncchd.go.jp (H.N.); tajima-g@ncchd.go.jp (G.T.)
* Correspondence: yosuke@u-fukui.ac.jp; Tel.: +81-776-61-3111; Fax: +81-776-61-8129

Abstract: To minimize false-positive cases in newborn screening by tandem mass spectrometry in Japan, practical second-tier liquid chromatography-tandem mass spectrometry analyses have been developed using a multimode ODS column with a single set of mobile phases and different gradient elution programs specific to the analysis of acylcarnitines, acylglycines, amino acids, and organic acids. Most analyses were performed using underivatized samples, except for analysis of methylcitric acid, and careful conditioning of the column was necessary for analyses of organic acids. Our second-tier tests enabled us to measure many metabolites useful for detection of target disorders, including allo-isoleucine, homocysteine, methylmalonic acid, and methylcitric acid. We found that accumulation of 3-hydroxyglutaric acid was specific to glutaric acidemia type I and that the ratio of 3-hydroxyisovaleric acid to 3-hydroxyisovalerylcarnitine was useful to detect newborns of mothers with 3-methylcrotonyl-CoA carboxylase deficiency. Data from the analysis of short-chain acylcarnitine and acylglycine were useful for differential diagnosis in cases positive for C5-OH-acylcarnitine or C5-acylcarnitine.

Keywords: isomer; stable-isotope dilution; derivatization; homocystinuria; cobalamin; biotin; maternal 3-methylcronylglycinuria; argininosuccinic acid

1. Introduction

In newborn screening using dried blood spots (DBSs) and flow-injection tandem mass spectrometry (MS/MS) in Japan, a series of acylcarnitines and amino acids, such as valine, leucine (Leu)+isoleucine (Ile), methionine (Met), phenylalanine, and citrulline, have been measured for the screening of fatty acid oxidation disorders, organic acidemias, maple syrup urine disease (MSUD), phenylketonuria, homocystinuria, and citrullinemia, and the recall rates have been relatively high, considering the proposed value [1]. In 2017, 946,065 newborns were born in Japan, and the overall official recall rate was 0.31%, with recall rates of 0.074% for propionylcarnitine (C3), 0.065% for pentanoylcarnitines (C5), 0.009% for hydroxypentanoylcarnitines (C5-OH), 0.055% for pentadioylcarnitines (C5-DC), 0.033% for Leu+Ile, 0.005% for Met, and 0.009% for citrulline. In cases of positive results for screening markers for fatty acid oxidation disorders, serum samples instead of DBSs are analyzed before diagnostic tests such as enzyme assays or gene analyses.

Catabolic conditions in newborns, such as in those who were fed poorly owing to strict breastfeeding, which has been often controversial in Japan, can yield false-positive results in screening for MSUD, glutaric acidemia type I (GA1), carnitine palmitoyltransferase-2 deficiency, and very-long chain acyl-CoA dehydrogenase deficiency in Japan. In addition,

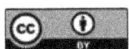

false-positive results may be due to low ability to discriminate among isomers of acylcarnitines and amino acids by flow-injection MS/MS. Although allo-isoleucine (allo-Ile) has been reported to be a sensitive disease marker [2–5] in MSUD screening, allo-Ile values cannot be obtained by flow-injection MS/MS measurement. In GA1, C5-DC is not thought to be a reliable marker for GA1 because the value of C5-DC in flow-injection MS/MS measurement consists of glutarylcarnitine and 3-hydroxyhexanoylcarnitine, both of which are accumulated in a catabolic state, whereas 3-hydroxyglutaric acid (3HGA) in plasma and urine is thought to be a useful diagnostic marker [6–9].

C3 and C3/C2 are classical screening markers for propionic acidemia (PAE) and a group of methylmalonic acidemias (MMAEs), including defects in cobalamin metabolism and maternal cobalamin deficiency. In the latter disease, C3 values tend to be lower than the traditional cut-offs for PAE and MMAE. We have experienced a false-negative case with cblD who developed MMAE without homocystinuria after viral enteritis in infancy and false-negative cases with cobalamin deficiency, which forced us to adopt lower cut-offs for C3 and C3/C2 and additional screening markers of C3/Met ratio and Met, the latter of which is necessary for methylene tetrahydrofolate reductase deficiency (MTHFRD) screening [10,11]. To detect these disorders, methylmalonic acid (MMA), methyl-citric acid (MCA), 3-hydroxypropionic acid (3HPA), and total homocysteine (tHcy) in DBSs measured by liquid chromatography (LC)-MS/MS have been reported to be powerful disease markers [12–17].

C5 is used as a screening marker for isovaleric acidemia (IVAE) and consists of such isomers as isovalerylcarnitine (IVC), valerylcarnitine, 2-methylbutyrylcarnitine (MBC), and pivaloylcarnitine. Positive results for C5 are suggestive of IVAE and 2-methylbutyryl-CoA dehydrogenase deficiency and can occur following the administration of pivaloyl group-containing drugs; moreover, LC-MS/MS analysis of these isomers is useful for differential diagnosis [18–20].

Citrulline is a screening marker for argininosuccinic acid synthetase deficiency, argininosuccinic acid lyase deficiency, and citrin deficiency. For the differential diagnosis of these disorders, argininosuccinic acid is measured in DBSs [5].

C5-OH is a screening marker for 3-methylcrotonyl-CoA carboxylase deficiency (3MCCD), multiple carboxylase deficiency, biotin deficiency, 3-hydroxy-3-methylglutaryl-CoA lyase deficiency (HMGLD), and 3-ketothiolase deficiency (KTD), and, in the traditional scheme, additional urinary organic acid analysis using gas chromatography-MS is necessary for differential diagnosis. In these disorders, acylcarnitines, including tiglylcarnitine in plasma, are measured by LC-MS/MS [21], and disease markers, such as tiglylglycine, methylcrotonyl-glycine (MCG), 3-hydroxyisoveleric acid (HIVA), 3-hydroxy-3-methylglutaric acid (HMGA), and 3-hydroxy-2-methylbutyrylcarnitine (HMBC) in DBSs, are thought to be useful.

Although the above-mentioned LC-MS/MS analyses of the disease markers in DBSs may have promising applications in decreasing recall rates [10,11], different measurement conditions have been reported from various laboratories using different LC columns. In the current study, we developed LC-MS/MS methods to measure many types of marker in DBSs using a single LC column and a single set of mobile phases.

2. Materials and Methods
2.1. Materials
2.1.1. Biological Samples

DBSs from patients were prepared during the newborn period for mass screening using MS/MS and then stored in a refrigerator in screening laboratories. Samples were then transported to our laboratory at the University of Fukui and measured using LC-MS/MS after obtaining permission from the parents of each patient. Diagnoses for patients with the target disorders in newborn screening were confirmed by enzyme or gene analysis. A patient with tyrosinemia type I was transferred to University of Fukui Hospital because of liver failure at 5 months of age, and succinylacetone levels in DBSs and urine were measured during treatments.

2.1.2. Chemicals

A NeoSMAAT kit for MS/MS newborn screening, which contains labeled acyl-carnitines and amino acids, was purchased from Sekisui Medical Co. (Tokyo, Japan). Methylmalonic acid-d_3, homocysteine-d_4, methylcitric acid, methylcitric acid-d_3, and argininosuccinic acid-$^{13}C_6 \cdot ^{15}N_4$ were purchased from Cambridge Isotope Laboratories (Andover, MA, USA); glutaric acid-d_4, 3-hydroxyglutaric acid, 3-hydroxyglutaric acid-d_4, and succinylacetone-$^{13}C_4$ were purchased from the VU Medical Center Metabolic Laboratory (Amsterdam, The Netherlands); 3-hydroxy-3-methylglutaric acid-d_3, methylcrotonylglycine-d_2, tiglylglycine-d_2, and propionylglycine-d_2 were purchased from CDN Isotope (Point-Claire, Canada); 3-hydroxypropionic acid, 3-hydroxyisovaleric acid, 3-hydroxy-3-methylglutaric acid, pivaloyl chloride, and succinylacetone were purchased from Tokyo Chemical Industry (Tokyo, Japan); 3-hydroxy-2-methylbutyric acid was purchased from Santa Cruz Biotechnology (Dallas, TX, USA); 2-hydroxyglutaric acid was purchased from Toronto Research Chemicals (Toronto, ON, Canada); and allo-Ile was purchased from Wako Chemicals (Kyoto, Japan). Pivaloylcarnitine was synthesized in our laboratory using pivaloyl chloride [18].

2.2. Methods

LC-MS/MS measurements for metabolites related to screening markers listed in Table 1 were performed.

Table 1. LC-MS/MS methods for the metabolites related to the screening markers.

LC-MS/MS Method	Positive Screening Marker	Target Metabolite
1	Leu+Ile	allo-Ile, Ile, Leu
2-A	C3, C3/C2, Met	MMA, 3HPA, tHcy
2-B	C3, C3/C2, Met	MMA, MCA, tHcy (derivatized)
3	C5-DC	GA, 3HGA
4	C5-OH, C5:1	HIVA, HMGA, HMBA
5	C5-OH, C5:1	short-chain acylcarnitines, acylglycines
6	C5	short-chain acylcarnitines
7	citrulline	argininosuccinic acid

For FI-MS/MS or LC-MS/MS analysis of acylcarnitines and amino acids, one punch-out (1/8 inch diameter) of a DBS was extracted using 100 µL methanol solution of the NeoSMAAT internal standard kit for routine methods for newborn screening, which contains leucine (5 µM), propionylcarnitine-d_3 (0.075 µM), isovalerylcarnitine-d_9 (0.075 µM), and 3-hydroxyisovalerylcarnitine-d_9 (0.075 µM). After FI-MS/MS analysis, positive samples were analyzed by LC-MS/MS with addition of 2% formic acid water/methanol (1:1) to the plate well.

For analysis of acylcarnitines and acylglycins, one punch-out of a DBS was extracted using 100 µL methanol solution from the NeoSMAAT kit spiked with labeled acylglycines as internal standards: propionylglycine-d_2 (1.53 µM), tiglylglycine-d_2 (1.27 µM), and 3-methylcrotonylglycine-d_2 (1.27 µM).

Total homocysteine and related organic acids were measured according to reported methods [11] with some modifications. The mixture from one punch-out of a DBS and 150 µL reaction solution (acetonitrile/distilled water/formic acid = 59:41:0.42) containing di-thio-threitol (0.77 mg), methylmalonic acid-d_3 (1.19 µM), homocysteine-d_4 (0.90 µM), and methylcitric acid-d_3 (0.69 µM) in a test tube was shaken slowly (120 rpm) at 25 °C for 60 min, and the supernatant was collected after centrifugation. The supernatant was dried under a nitrogen stream and was redissolved in a 2% formic acid water/methanol solution (1:1). For measurement of derivatized samples, the dried extract was derivatized with butanol·HCl at 65 °C for 25 min, dried again, and redissolved in 2% formic acid water/methanol solution (1:1).

For analysis of GA and 3HGA, one punch-out of a DBS was extracted using 100 µL 98% methanol solution containing glutaric acid-d_4 (0.38 µM) and 3-hydroxyglutaric acid-d_4 (0.33 µM) as internal standards. For analysis of HIVA, HMGA and HMBA, one punch-out of a DBS was extracted using 100 µL 98% methanol solution containing 3-hydroxy-3-methylglutaric acid-d_3 (0.30 µM). For analysis of argininosuccinic acid, one punch-out of a DBS was extracted using 100 µL of 90% methanol solution containing argininosuccinic acid-$^{13}C_6 \cdot ^{15}N_4$ (1.67 µM). For analysis of succinylacetone, the mixture of one punch-out of a DBS and 110 µL of 80% aceto-nitril solution containing succinylacetone-$^{13}C_4$ (0.20 µM), 0.1% hydrazine H_2O, and 0.1% formic acid was stirred slowly for 45 min, and the supernatant was collected after centrifugation. The extract was dried under a nitrogen stream and redissolved in 2% formic acid water/methanol solution (1:1).

The samples (10 µL) were introduced into the LC mobile phase flow (flow rate: 0.4 mL/min) using a 150 mm × 3.0 mm Scherzo SS-C18 column (Imtakt, Portland, OR, USA). Gradient elution of the analytes was achieved using a program with mobile phase A (aqueous 0.5% formic acid) and mobile phase B ((0.5 M ammonium formate/0.5 M NH_4OH = 9:1)/methanol = 1:9), as detailed in the legends for the corresponding Figures.

For measurements using electrospray-ionization LC-MS/MS, a model API 4000 triple-stage mass spectrometer (AB Sciex, Tokyo, Japan) equipped with a model LC10Avp HPLC system and a model SIL-20AC auto-injector (Shimadzu, Kyoto, Japan) was used [21]. The MS/MS analyses were performed in multiple reaction monitoring (MRM) mode using the transitions detailed in the Figures. Underivatized organic acids were analyzed in negative ion mode. Suitable measurement conditions for the designated transitions were identified with the automatic tune function in Analyst software. For quantification, the recorded peak area of the designated MRM ion set was used.

Allo-Ile was quantified using leucine-d_3 as an internal standard instead of stable isotope-labeled allo-Ile. The aqueous calibrator for the calibration curve contained 16.7, 83.3, 166.6, or 333.3 µM allo-Ile. Based on the assumption that one punch-out (1/8 inch diameter) of a DBS contains 3 µL whole blood, the mixture of 3 µL of the calibrator and 100 µL internal standard solution from the NeoSMAAT internal standard kit was analyzed to determine the linearity. In the mixture, the concentration of allo-Ile was 0.1×, 0.5×, 1×, or 2× that of leucine-d_3.

Similarly, pivaloylcarnitine was quantified using isovalerylcarnitine-d_9 as an internal standard instead of stable isotope-labeled pivaloylcarnitine. The calibrator for the calibration curve contained 0.25, 1.25, 2.5, or 5.0 µM pivaloylcarnitine, and the mixture of 3 µL the calibrator and 100 µL the internal standard solution from the NeoSMAAT internal standard kit was analyzed.

HIVA and HMBA were quantified using 3-hydroxy-3-methylglutaric acid-d_3 as an internal standard. The calibrator for calibration curve contained 1.0, 5.0, 10.0, or 20.0 µM HMGA, HIVA, and HMBA, and the mixture of 3 µL calibrator and 100 µL internal standard solution was analyzed.

To determine the linearity of analyses other than allo-Ile, pivaloylcarnitine, HIVA and HMBA, we also analyzed the mixture of calibrator and internal standard, in which the target metabolite level was 0.1×, 0.5×, 1×, or 2× that of the internal standard. Intra- and inter-assay imprecisions were tested by analysis of patient DBSs.

3. Results

In analyses using the stable isotope dilution method with the stable isotope-labeled compound as an internal standard, the calibration curves were linear in the test concentration range. Intra- and inter-assay CV values in analyses of patient DBSs were less than 10%, except for those of HIVA and HMBA assays.

An LC-MS/MS chromatogram of the allo-Ile measurement using a DBS from a newborn with MSUD is shown in Figure 1. Allo-Ile concentrations in DBSs were calculated based on a calibration curve using the aqueous solutions of allo-Ile and leucine-d_3, which was linear (R^2 = 0.9994) up to an allo-Ile concentration corresponding to 333.3 µM in DBS.

Those of patients with MSUD are listed in Table 2, together with those in false-positive cases. Intra-assay CV (n = 5) and inter-assay CV (n = 5) were 5.4% and 8.1%, respectively, at an allo-Ile concentration of 38.3 µM in DBS.

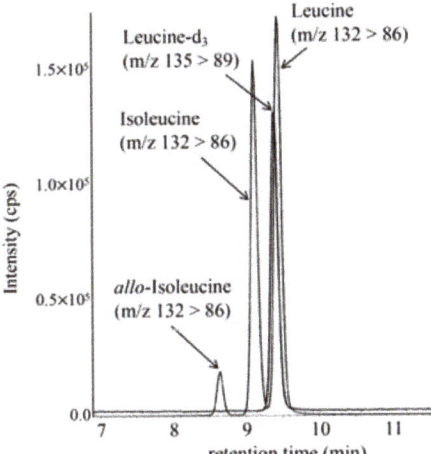

Figure 1. LC-MS/MS analysis of allo-Ile was performed using the following gradient elution program: 20% B (0.1 min), 20% to 30% B (3 min), 30% to 51% B (7 min), 51% to 100% B (0.1 min), 100% B (7.9 min), 100% to 20% B (0.1 min), and 20% B (5 min), with a flow rate of 0.3 mL/min.

Table 2. Allo-Ile, related amino acid, and acetylcarnitine levels (µM) in patients with maple syrup urine disease, as measured by LC-MS/MS.

MSUD Patient #	FI-MS/MS			LC-MS/MS
	Acetylcarnitine	Valine	Leu+Ile	Allo-Ile
1	40.7	368	767	38.3
2	20.5	427	554	82.1
3	15.0	386	2199	362.6
4	17.9	508	813	131.0
false positive cases (n = 12)	15.0–38.2	211–420	304–420	0.5–5.9

LC-MS/MS chromatograms for analyses of MMA, MCA, and tHcy in DBSs from a newborn with cobalamin deficiency type C (cblC), using an underivatized sample (A) and a derivatized sample (B), are shown in Figure 2. In our analysis of underivatized samples, the peaks of MCA did not show good quality, although this was obtained for the analysis of derivatized samples. In the analysis of derivatized samples, 3HPA concentrations could not be measured well, likely owing to the low ionization efficiency of 3HPA-butylester and sample loss during preparation.

In derivatized sample measurements from control newborns (n = 13), the concentrations of MMA, MCA, and tHcy ranged from 0.20 to 0.99 µM, 0.20 (below the detection limit) to 0.75 µM, and 1.1 to 4.9 µM, respectively. In patients with MMAE, including cblA and cblD (n = 8), MMA concentrations ranged from 15.0 to 863.9 µM. MCA concentrations obtained from derivatized sample measurements in patients with PAE (n = 13) ranged from 0.92 to 3.50 µM, whereas 3HPA concentrations obtained from underivatized sample measurements in patients with PAE (n = 13) and control newborns ranged from 9.6 to 32.8 µM and 1.7 to 8.8 µM, respectively.

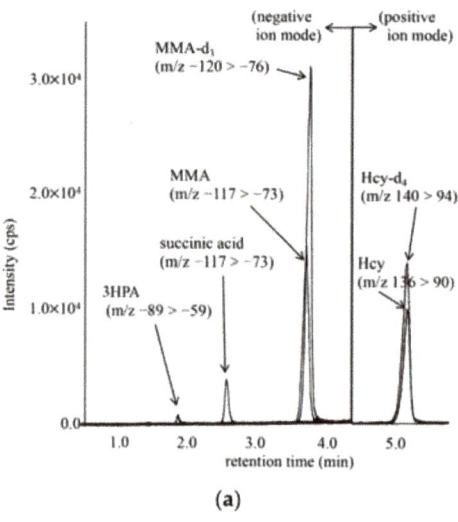 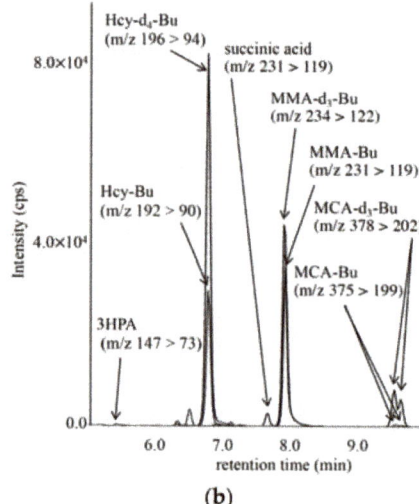

Figure 2. LC-MS/MS analysis of underivatized organic acids, including methylmalonic acid (MMA) using negative ion mode and homocysteine (Hcy) by positive ion mode (**a**), and that for derivatized organic acids, including methylcitric acid butyl-ester (MCA-Bu) and Hcy butyl-ester (Hcy-Bu) by positive ion mode (**b**). The gradient elution program in (**a**) was as follows: 13% B (0.5 min), 13% to 30% B (6 min), 30% to 100% B (0.1 min), 100% B (7.9 min), 100% to 10% B (0.1 min), and 13% B (5 min); that in (**b**) was as follows: 0% B (0.2 min), 0% to 80% B (1 min), 80% to 100% B (9 min), 100% B (3 min), 100% to 0% B (0.1 min), and 0% B (3 min).

In underivatized sample measurements, MMA and tHcy concentrations in patients with cblC, maternal cobalamin-deficiency, MFHFRD, and CBSD are shown in Table 3. These patients were characterized by elevated tHcy concentrations.

Table 3. Methylmalonic acid (MMA) and total homocysteine (tHcy) in DBSs of patients with positive results in screening markers of C3 (propionylcarnitine), C3/C2, C3/Met, and Met (methionine).

Pt #	Diagnosis	FI-MS/MS				LC-MS/MS	
		C3 (μM)	C3/C2	C3/Met	Met (μM)	MMA (μM)	tHcy (μM)
1	cblC	10.30	1.10	1.60	6.40	59.7	34.8
2	cblC	15.01	1.10	0.46	32.5	44.4	17.0
3	cobalamin deficiency [1]	3.59	0.21	0.34	10.65	6.7	5.5
4	cobalamin deficiency [1]	2.14	0.45	0.35	6.12	5.5	11.8
5	MTHFRD	0.62	0.13	0.13	4.98	0.5	49.2
6	MTHFRD	0.45	0.05	0.07	6.63	0.8	10.6
7	MTHFRD	0.77	0.09	0.17	4.61	1.3	10.4
8	MTHFRD	0.53	0.09	0.08	6.70	0.8	28.7
9	CBSD [2]	1.00	0.02	0.00	911	0.1	84.7
	upper cut-off	3.5	0.25	0.25	80	1.0	5.0
	lower cut-off	-	-	-	9.27	-	-

[1] The infants with cobalamin-deficiency were born to mothers with ileum-resection and chronic atrophic gastritis, and were exclusively breast-fed for several months and developed symptoms. The values were obtained using their DBSs for newborn screening which were stored in refrigerators. [2] cystathionine beta-synthase deficiency.

LC-MS/MS chromatogram for analysis of GA and 3HGA in the DBS from a newborn with GA1 is shown in Figure 3. 3HGA was quantified based on a transition that was different from that of 2-hydroxyglutaric acid. The concentrations of 3HGA in newborn DBSs from three patients ranged from 1.08 to 1.44 μM (mean ± standard deviation in controls: 0.35 ± 0.10), and those of glutaric acid (GA) ranged from 12.1 to 25.8 µM (in controls: 6.67 ± 2.95).

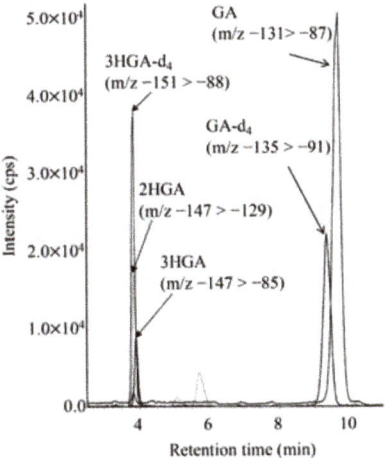

Figure 3. LC-MS/MS analysis for underivatized glutaric acid (GA), 3-hydroxyglutaric acid (3HGA), and 2-hydroxyglutaric acid (2HGA) using negative ion mode. The gradient elution program was as follows: 0% B (5 min), 0% to 30% B (6 min), 30% to 100% B (0.1 min), 100% B (7.9 min), 100% to 10% B (0.1 min), and 13% B (5 min).

LC-MS/MS chromatograms for analyses of HMG, HIVA, and HMBA in the DBS of a newborn with KTD are shown in Figure 4. The concentrations of HIVA and HMBA were calculated based on the calibration curves using the aqueous solutions of HIVA, HMBA and HMGA-d_3. The calibration curves were linear, and intra- and inter-assay CV values in analyses of patient DBSs are given in Table 4.

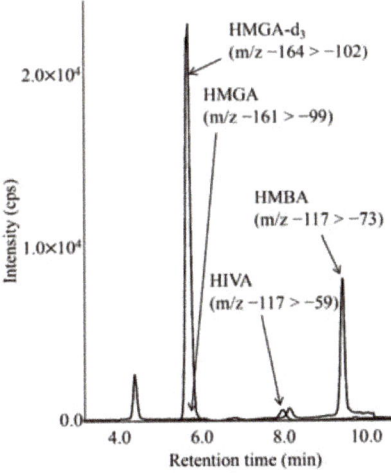

Figure 4. LC-MS/MS analysis for underivatized 3-hydroxy-3-methylglutaric acid (HMGA) and 3-hydroxyisovaleric acid (HIVA) using negative ion mode. The gradient elution program was as follows: 0% B (5 min), 0% to 38% B (6 min), 38% to 100% B (0.1 min), 100% B (5.9 min), 100% to 0% B (0.1 min), and 0% B (5 min).

Table 4. Assay validation for HMGA, HIVA, and HMBA analysis.

Analyte	Linearity (R^2)	Analyte Level in DBS (μM)	Imprecision	
			CV (%) Intraassay (n = 5)	CV (%) Inter-assay (n = 5)
HMGA	0.9994	5.1	5.1	7.9
HIVA	0.9982	14.7	7.6	12.2
HMBA	0.9974	39.1	8.9	14.4

LC-MS/MS chromatograms for analyses of acylcarnitines and acylglycines in DBSs from a newborn with KTD (a) and a newborn with 3MCCD (b) are shown in Figure 5. In KTD, increased tiglylcarnitine, tiglylglycine, and 3-hydroxy-2-methylbutyrylcarnitine levels were observed, whereas increased 3-methylcrotonylglycine and 3-hydroxyisovalerylcarnitine (HIVC) levels were characteristic in 3MCCD. The MRM transition of m/z 262 > 145, in addition to that of 262 > 85, was used for measurement of 3-hydroxyisovalerylcarnitine, since complete chromatographic separation between 3-hydroxyisovalerylcarnitine and 3-hydroxy-2-methylbutyrylcarnitine (HMBC) was not achieved [21].

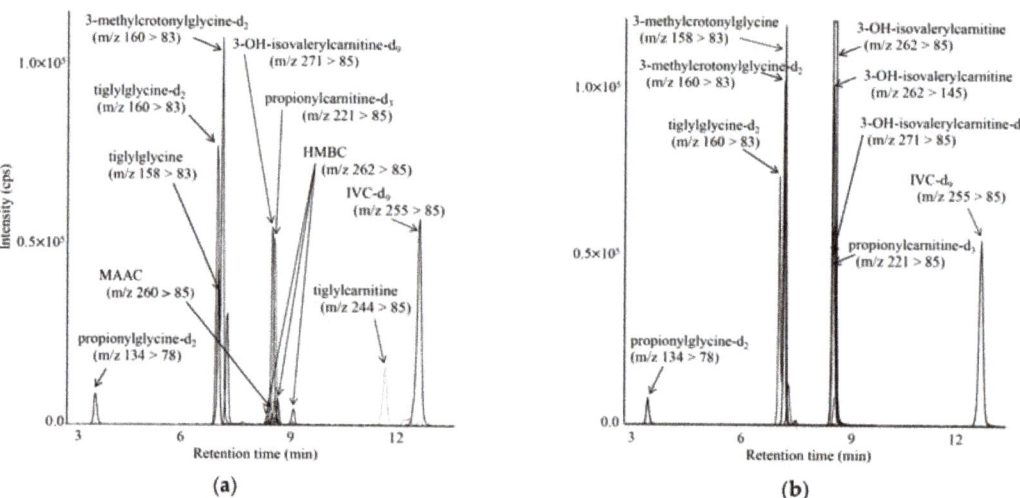

Figure 5. LC-MS/MS analyses for propionylglycine, tiglylglycine, and 3-methylcrotonylglycine, together with acylcarnitines, including tiglylcarnitine, using positive ion mode for a newborn with KTD (a) and a newborn with 3MCCD (b). The gradient elution program was as follows: 10% B (1 min), 10% to 40% B (4 min), 40% to 59% B (9 min), 55% to 100% B (0.1 min), 100% B (6.9 min), 100% to 10% B (0.1 min), and 10% B (5 min).

Metabolites in patients with diseases characterized by high C5-OH-acylcarnitine concentrations are listed in Table 5. 3-Ketothiolase deficiency was characterized by elevated 3-hydroxy-2-methylbutyric acid (HMBA), 3-hydroxy-2-methylbutyrylcarnitine (HMBC), and tiglylglycine; HMGLD was characterized by elevated HMGA; holo-carboxylase deficiency was characterized by elevated HIVA, HIVC, and propionylglycine; and 3MCCD was characterized by elevated HIVA, HIVC, and 3-methylcrotonylglycine. In babies born to mothers with 3MCCD, the ratios of HIVA to HIVC (0.2–2.9) were markedly lower than those (23.8, 79.9) in patients with 3MCCD.

Table 5. Organic acids, acylcarnitines, and acylglycines in DBSs from newborns with high C5-OH levels.

Diagnosis	FI-MS/MS	LC-MS/MS										
	C5-OH (µM)	Organic Acid (µM)			Acylcarnitine (µM)					Acylglycine (µM)		
		HMGA	HIVA	3HMBA	Propionyl	HIVC	HMBC	Tiglyl	MCC [1]	Propionyl	Tiglyl	MCG [2]
3-ketothiolase deficiency	3.1	0.37	2.2	130.3	0.67	0.12	4.84	0.49	<0.01	0.02	2.67	0.01
	2.8	0.10	1.3	39.1	1.62	0.13	3.61	0.62	<0.01	0.09	4.10	<0.01
HMGLD	3.1	5.19	25.3	0.66	0.19	2.78	0.01	0.01	<0.01	0.04	0.01	0.07
Holo-carboxylase deficiency	2.2	1.04	624.5	0.44	1.78	1.44	0.02	0.03	<0.01	1.49	0.26	2.10
	3.4	0.19	187.5	0.53	4.12	3.35	0.01	<0.01	0.01	0.73	0.02	0.91
mild biotin deficiency	1.1	0.04	5.8	0.11	0.81	1.09	0.01	<0.01	<0.01	0.01	0.01	0.04
3MCCD	11.9	0.23	238.5	0.60	0.13	10.01	0.01	<0.01	<0.01	0.01	0.01	3.66
	3.4	0.45	326.6	0.47	0.85	4.09	0.01	<0.01	0.01	0.03	0.01	1.08
	6.8	0.11	14.7	0.39	0.41	5.10	0.01	<0.01	<0.01	0.02	0.03	0.43
Baby born to mother with 3MCCD	3.9	0.24	11.7	0.55	0.86	5.69	0.01	<0.01	<0.01	0.02	0.02	0.01
	4.8	0.06	1.0	0.20	0.39	4.54	0.06	<0.01	<0.01	0.01	0.01	0.01
controls (mean ± SD)	<0.5	0.53 ± 0.20	2.1 ± 0.6	0.60 ± 0.11	1.17 ± 0.45	0.09 ± 0.03	<0.01	<0.01	<0.01	0.02 ± 0.01	0.01 ± 0.01	<0.01

[1] 3-methylcrotonylcarnitine, [2] 3-methylcrotonylglycine.

LC-MS/MS chromatogram for analysis of short-chain acylcarnitines in the DBS from a newborn treated with antibiotics is shown in Figure 6. The peaks of 3 isomers appeared separately, and the condition was characterized by increased pivaloylcarnitine concentrations, which were calculated based on a calibration curve using aqueous solutions of pivaloylcarnitine and isovalerylcarnitine-d_9. The calibration curve was linear ($R^2 = 0.9995$) up to the pivaloylcarnitine concentration corresponding to 5.5 µM in DBS. Intra-assay CV (n = 5) and inter-assay CV (n = 5) for pivaloylcarnitine were 4.2% and 9.2%, respectively, at a pivaloylcarnitine concentration of 3.7 µM in DBS. Concentrations of pivaloylcarnitine and IVC in control newborns (n = 13) were below the detection limit (0.01 µM) and 0.17 ± 0.10 µM, respectively. Those of pivaloylcarnitine in newborns treated with antibiotics ranged 1.2 to 9.7 µM, and those of IVC in patients with isovaleric acidemia ranged from 1.5 to 17.2 µM.

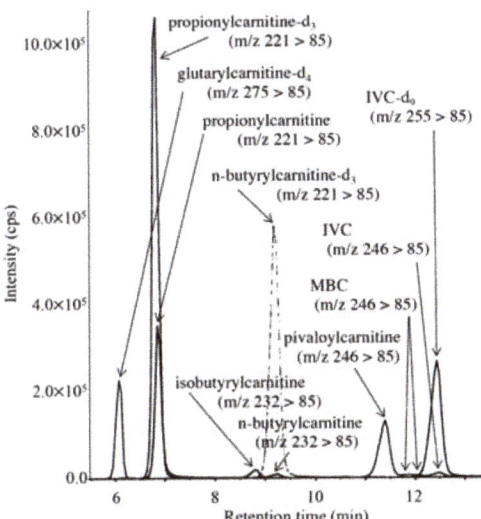

Figure 6. LC-MS/MS analysis for pivaloylcarnitine, 2-methylbutyrylcarnitine, isovalerylcarnitine, n-butyrylcarnitine, and isobutyrylcarnitine. The gradient elution program was as follows: 10% B (1 min), 10% to 40% B (4 min), 40% to 70% B (8 min), 70% to 100% B (0.1 min), 100% B (6.9 min), and 100% to 10% B (0.1 min).

LC-MS/MS chromatograms for analyses of argininosuccinic acid in DBSs of a newborn with argininesuccinate lyase deficiency and a control newborn are shown in Figure 7. The limit of quantification was 0.05 nmol/mL in DBSs.

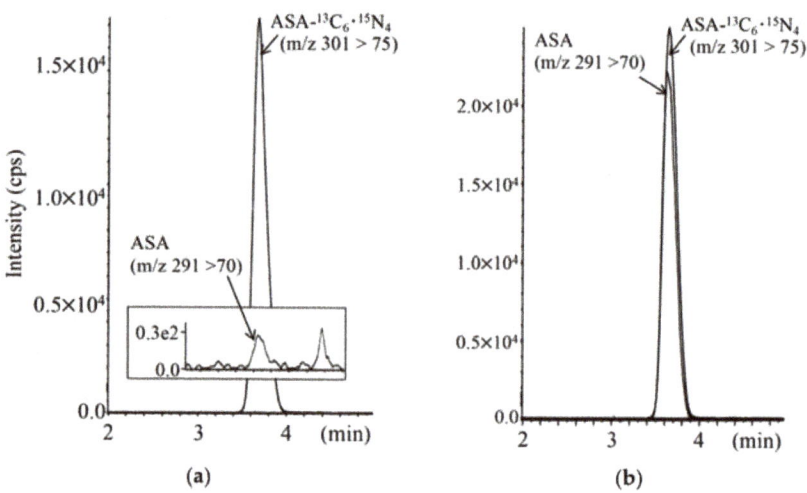

Figure 7. LC-MS/MS analysis for argininosuccinic acid (ASA) using positive ion mode for a control newborn (**a**) and a newborn with argininesuccinate lyase deficiency (**b**). The gradient elution program was as follows: 0% B (1 min), 0% to 30% B (4 min), 30% to 100% B (0.5 min), 100% B (5.5 min), 100% to 10% B (0.5 min), and 10% B (5 min).

LC-MS/MS chromatogram for analysis of succinylacetone in the DBS from a patient with tyrosinemia type 1 is shown in Figure 8, together with the clinical course and succinylacetone concentrations for the patient. The succinylacetone concentration in the newborn DBS stored in a refrigerator for 5 months was 28.7 nmol/mL, whereas that in control newborn DBSs was 0.21 ± 0.10 nmol/mL.

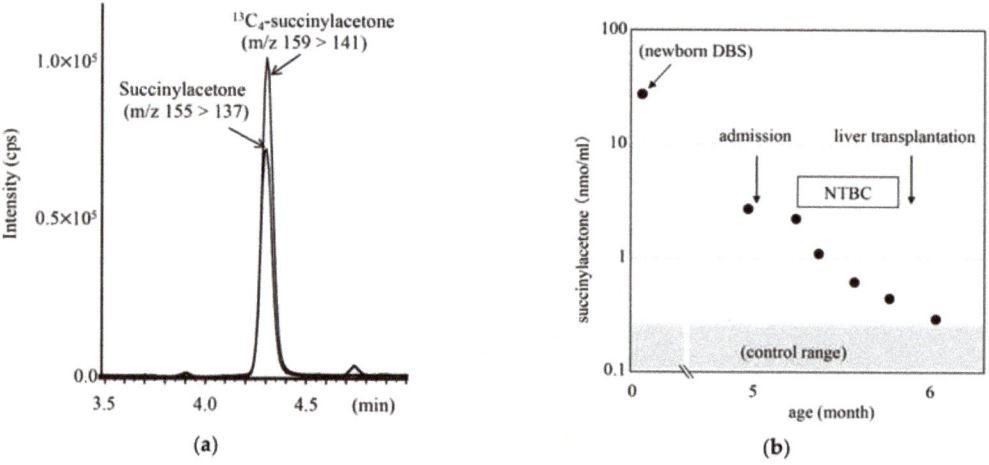

Figure 8. LC-MS/MS analysis for succinylacetone (SA) using positive ion mode (**a**) and clinical course of a patient with tyrosinemia type 1 (**b**). Gradient elution program: 20% B (0.1 min), 20% to 100% B (5 min), 100% B (5 min), 100% to 20% B (0.5 min), and 20% B (4 min).

4. Discussion

To manage positive cases with screening markers such as C3, C5, C5-OH, C5-DC, Leu+Ile, Met, and citrulline, we developed practical second-tier tests using a single LC column and a single set of mobile phases together with different gradient elution programs specific for the designated LC-MS/MS measurements. We used a multimode ODS Scherzo SS-C18 column with anion and cation exchange and showed excellent chromatographic ability for amino acids, short- to medium-chain acylcarnitines, and acylglycines. In addition, our methods for acylcarnitines and allo-Ile analysis were convenient because the positive samples could be measured in wells of a plate following addition of 2% formic acid/methanol for our second-tier LC-MS/MS.

Despite these advancements, LC-MS/MS measurements of organic acids are still challenging. Organic acids with multiple carboxyl groups are difficult to analyze using underivatized samples [13], and analytical methods for derivatized samples have been adopted in several laboratories [11,14]. However, analysis of butylated organic acids may still be difficult owing to the relatively poor ionization efficiency in electrospray-ionization or the high volatility of small molecule organic acids. Because MS/MS measurements of organic acids are performed in negative mode, whereas those of amino acids are performed in positive mode, MS/MS instruments with the ability to switch quickly between the two modes are needed for measurement of both organic acids and amino acids when using underivatized samples. Moreover, some stable isotope-labeled organic acids are not available from reagent manufacturers.

In the current study, using underivatized samples, MCA could not be quantified, and 3HPA was measured using methylmalonic acid-d_3 as an internal standard because stable isotope-labeled 3HPA was not available. Nevertheless, 3HPA levels in our underivatized sample measurements were found to be useful for practical detection of mild PAE. Next, we used methods for sample preparation and derivatization for analyses of MMA, MCA, and tHcy [11], which enabled us to achieve practical LC-MS/MS analysis using our mobile phases for the SS-C18 column. MCA levels obtained with this measurement approach were useful for detection of PAE.

Preferably, LC-MS/MS analysis should be performed using underivatized samples because time-consuming sample preparation processes may result in damage to analytes. In addition, derivatization can be challenging because of the need for a fume hood and drying apparatus in screening laboratories. LC-MS/MS measurement of tHcy together with MMA is useful for screening of a series of homo-cystinurias [11]. In our system, measurement of tHcy and MMA could be performed using both derivatized and underivatized samples. Indeed, our results for tHcy and MMA levels provided additional useful information in the screening of cblC, cobalamin deficiency, MTHFRD, and CBSD. In Japan, a pilot study of homocystinuria screening with modified cut-offs for C3 and C3/C2 and an additional marker of C3/Met is currently underway, combined with a second-tier test for MMA and tHcy measurement using underivatized samples.

Our LC-MS/MS measurements were based mostly on the stable isotope dilution technique. However, suitable stable isotope-labeled internal standards were not available for the quantification of some acylcarnitines, including tiglylcarnitine, pivaloylcarnitine, 2-methylbutyrylcarnitine, and 3-hydroxy-2-methylbutyrylcarnitine, although the values for these acylcarnitines, calculated using isovalerylcarnitine-d_9 as an internal standard, are practically precise in newborn screening. In contrast, measurements of organic acids, such as HIVA and 3HMBA, using 3-hydroxy-3-methylglutaric acid-d_3 as an internal standard, should be performed with careful conditioning of the column in order to obtain precise values. Notably, the ratio of HIVA to HIVC may be useful for identifying babies born to mothers with 3MCCD because the practice of identifying mothers with mild 3MCCD using elevated C5-OH in DBSs of newborns may be controversial.

Regarding LC-MS/MS measurement of organic acids, 3HGA appears to have an important role when screening for GA1. Although DBS levels of glutarylcarnitine and GA apparently overlap between patients with GA1 and control newborns, those of 3HGA in patients with GA1 were significantly higher than those in control newborns. The wide distribution of glutarylcarnitine and GA levels may be affected by catabolic conditions in control newborns.

For practical application of newborn screening projects, identification of patients as early as possible is thought to be essential for initiation of appropriate treatment based on the laboratory data specific to the disease. Thus, data measured by LC-MS/MS for the follow-up of patients have been obtained from several screening laboratories [3,8,17,22]. Our methods can be applied to serum sample measurements, and serum and DBS concentrations of metabolites, such as MMA, tHcy, 3HGA, allo-Ile, argininosuccinic acid, and succinylacetone, by LC-MS/MS have been provided to hospitals for patient follow-up from our laboratories. Argininosuccinic acid measurement was sufficiently sensitive in our measurements compared with previously reported methods [5] and was useful to discriminate argininesuccinate lyase deficiency from argininesuccinate synthetase deficiency and citrin deficiency, while the screening kits that allow us to discriminate these disorders are not used, since argininesuccinate lyase deficiency is quite rare in Japan. Moreover, argininosuccinic acid data are used for evaluating the effects of long-term treatment. Tyrosinemia type I is extremely rare and is not included in the list of target disorders for newborn screening in Japan, and succinylacetone data obtained using LC-MS/MS may be used for the follow-up of patients, as shown in Figure 8.

Unfortunately, our second-tier tests have not yet been used in most of the screening laboratories in Japan. In Japan, 872,683 babies were born in 2020, and samples from newborns were tested in 37 screening laboratories. In the majority of these laboratories, fewer than 10,000 newborns are tested annually using a single LC-MS/MS instrument, and LC-MS/MS measurements as second-tier tests seemed to be a significant burden to a limited number of staff, mainly because of the additional work required to maintain equipment performance, despite our simple measurement approach. Consolidation of screening work in a reduced number of laboratories and an additional LC-MS/MS instrument for second-tier tests, with some type of kit for quality assurance, including sufficient labeled internal standards, may facilitate the use of these tests in screening laboratories.

Author Contributions: Conceptualization, Y.S. and G.T.; Writing, Y.S.; Visualization, Y.S. and M.Y.; Methodology, Y.S., M.Y., N.I. and H.N.; Funding Acquisition, G.T. All authors have read and agreed to the published version of the manuscript.

Funding: This research was supported partly by The Grant of National Center for Child Health and Development (2020C-1).

Institutional Review Board Statement: This study was approved by the Institutional Ethics Committee at the University of Fukui (#20130055, #20180029).

Informed Consent Statement: Informed consent was obtained from all subjects involved in the study.

Data Availability Statement: The data used to support the findings of this study are available from the corresponding author upon request.

Conflicts of Interest: The authors declare no conflict of interest.

References

1. Rinaldo, P.; Zafari, S.; Tortorelli, S.; Matern, D. Making the case for objective performance metrics in newborn screening by tandem mass spectrometry. *Ment. Retard. Dev. Disabil. Res. Rev.* **2006**, *12*, 255–261. [CrossRef]
2. Wendel, U.; Langenbeck, U.; Seakin, J.W.T. Interrelation between the metabolism of L-isoleucine and L-allo-isoleucine in patients with maple syrup urine disease. *Pediatr. Res.* **1989**, *25*, 11–14. [CrossRef] [PubMed]
3. Oglesbee, D.; Sanders, K.A.; Lacey, J.M.; Magera, M.J.; Casetta, B.; Strauss, K.A.; Tortorelli, S.; Rinaldo, P.; Matern, D. Second-tier test for quantification of alloisoleucine and branched-chain amino acids in dried blood spots to improve newborn screening for maple syrup urine disease (MSUD). *Clin. Chem.* **2008**, *54*, 542–549. [CrossRef] [PubMed]
4. Alodaib, A.; Carpenter, K.; Wiley, V.; Sim, K.; Christodoulou, J.; Wilcken, B. An improved ultra performance liquid chromatography-tandem mass spectrometry method for the determination of alloisoleucine and branched chain amino acids in dried blood samples. *Ann. Clin. Biochem.* **2011**, *48*, 468–470. [CrossRef] [PubMed]

5. Griffin, C.; Ammous, Z.; Vancea, G.H.; Grahama, B.H.; Miller, M.J. Rapid quantification of underivatized alloisoleucine and argininosuccinate using mixed-mode chromatography with tandem mass spectrometry. *J. Chromatogr. B Anal. Technol. Biomed. Life Sci.* **2019**, *1128*, 121786. [CrossRef]
6. Moore, T.; Le, A.; Cowan, T.M. An improved LC-MS/MS method for the detection of classic and low excretor glutaric acidemia type 1. *J. Inherit. Metab. Dis.* **2012**, *35*, 431–435. [CrossRef]
7. Peng, M.; Fang, X.; Huang, Y.; Cai, Y.; Liang, C.; Lin, R.; Liu, L.J. Separation and identification of underivatized plasma acylcarnitine isomers using liquid chromatography-tandem mass spectrometry for the differential diagnosis of organic acidemias and fatty acid oxidation defects. *Chromatogr. A* **2013**, *1319*, 97–106. [CrossRef]
8. Simon, G.A.; Wierenga, A. Quantitation of plasma and urine 3-hydroxyglutaric acid, after separation from 2-hydroxyglutaric acid and other compounds of similar ion transition, by liquid chromatography-tandem mass spectrometry for the confirmation of glutaric aciduria type 1. *J. Chromatogr. B Anal. Technol. Biomed. Life Sci.* **2018**, *1097–1098*, 101–110. [CrossRef]
9. Al-Dirbashi, O.Y.; Kölker, S.; Ng, D.; Fisher, L.; Rupar, T.; Lepage, N.; Rashed, M.S.; Santa, T.; Goodman, S.I.; Geraghty, M.T.; et al. Diagnosis of glutaric aciduria type 1 by measuring 3-hydroxyglutaric acid in dried urine spots by liquid chromatography tandem mass spectrometry. *J. Inherit. Metab. Dis.* **2011**, *34*, 173–180. [CrossRef]
10. Matern, D.; Tortorelli, S.; Oglesbee, D.; Gavrilov, D.; Rinaldo, P. Reduction of the false-positive rate in newborn screening by implementation of MS/MS-based second-tier tests: The MayoClinic experience (2004–2007). *J. Inherit. Metab. Dis.* **2007**, *30*, 585–592. [CrossRef]
11. Turgeon, C.T.; Magera, M.J.; Cuthbert, C.D.; Loken, P.R.; Gavrilov, D.K.; Tortorelli, S.; Raymond, K.M.; Oglesbee, D.; Rinaldo, P.; Matern, D. Determination of total homocysteine, methylmalonic acid, and 2-methylcitric acid in dried blood spots by tandem mass spectrometry. *Clin. Chem.* **2010**, *56*, 1686–1695. [CrossRef]
12. la Marca, G.; Malvagia, S.; Pasquini, E.; Innocenti, M.; Donati, M.A.; Zammarchi, E. Rapid 2nd-tier test for measurement of 3-OH-propionic and methylmalonic acids on dried blood spots: Reducing the false-positive rate for propionylcarnitine during expanded newborn screening by liquid chromatography-tandem mass spectrometry. *Clin. Chem.* **2007**, *53*, 1364–1369. [CrossRef]
13. Fu, X.; Xu, Y.K.; Chan, P.; Pattengale, P.K. Simple, fast, and simultaneous detection of plasma total homocysteine, methylmalonic acid, methionine, and 2-methylcitric acid using liquid chromatography and mass spectrometry (LC/MS/MS). *JIMD Rep.* **2013**, *10*, 69–78.
14. Al-Dirbashi, O.Y.; McIntosh, N.; McRoberts, C.; Fisher, L.; Rashed, M.S.; Makhseed, N.; Geraghty, M.T.; Santa, T.; Chakraborty, P. Analysis of methylcitrate in dried blood spots by liquid chromatography-tandem mass spectrometry. *JIMD Rep.* **2014**, *16*, 65–73. [PubMed]
15. Al-Dirbashi, O.Y.; McIntosh, N.; Chakraborty, P. Quantification of 2-methylcitric acid in dried blood spots improves newborn screening for propionic and methylmalonic acidemias. *J. Med. Screen* **2017**, *24*, 58–61. [CrossRef] [PubMed]
16. Monostori, P.; Klinke, G.; Richter, S.; Barath, A.; Fingerhut, R.; Baumgartner, M.R.; Kolker, S.; Hoffmann, G.F.; Gramer, G.; Okun, J.G. Simultaneous determination of 3-hydroxypropionic acid, methylmalonic acid and methylcitric acid in dried blood spots: Second-tier LC-MS/MS assay for newborn screening of propionic acidemia, methylmalonic acidemias and combined remethylation disorders. *PLoS ONE* **2017**, *12*, e0184897. [CrossRef] [PubMed]
17. Wang, Y.; Sun, Y.; Jiang, T. Clinical application of LC-MS/MS in the follow-up for treatment of children with methylmalonic aciduria. *Adv. Ther.* **2019**, *36*, 1304–1313. [CrossRef] [PubMed]
18. Nakajima, Y.; Ito, T.; Maeda, Y.; Ichiki, S.; Sugiyama, N.; Mizuno, M.; Makino, Y.; Sugiura, T.; Kurono, Y.; Togari, H. Detection of pivaloylcarnitine in pediatric patients with hypocarnitinemia after long-term administration of pivalate-containing antibiotics. *Tohoku J. Exp. Med.* **2010**, *221*, 309–313. [CrossRef] [PubMed]
19. Forni, S.; Fu, X.; Palmer, S.E.; Sweetman, L. Rapid determination of C4-acylcarnitine and C5-acylcarnitine isomers in plasma and dried blood spots by UPLC-MS/MS as a second tier test following flow-injection MS/MS acylcarnitine profile analysis. *Mol. Genet. Metab* **2010**, *101*, 25–32. [CrossRef]
20. Janzen, N.; Steuerwald, U.; Sander, S.; Terhardt, M.; Peter, M.; Sander, J. UPLC-MS/MS analysis of C5-acylcarnitines in dried blood spots. *Clin. Chim. Acta* **2013**, *421*, 41–45. [CrossRef] [PubMed]
21. Shigematsu, Y.; Yuasa, M.; Hata, I.; Nakajima, H.; Tajima, G.; Ishige, N.; Fukao, T.; Maeda, Y. 2-Methylacetoacetylcarnitine in blood of patients of beta-ketothiolase deficiency and HSD10 disease. *Med. Mass Spectrom.* **2019**, *3*, 43–47.
22. Maines, E.; Catesini, G.; Boenzi, S.; Mosca, A.; Candusso, M.; Strologo, L.D.; Martinelli, D.; Maiorana, A.; Liguori, A.; Olivieri, G.; et al. Plasma methylcitric acid and its correlations with other disease biomarkers: The impact in the follow up of patients with propionic and methylmalonic acidemia. *J. Inherit. Metab. Dis.* **2020**, *43*, 1173–1185. [CrossRef] [PubMed]

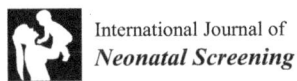

Review

Current Perspectives on Neonatal Screening for Propionic Acidemia in Japan: An Unexpectedly High Incidence of Patients with Mild Disease Caused by a Common *PCCB* Variant

Go Tajima [1,2,*], Reiko Kagawa [2], Fumiaki Sakura [2], Akari Nakamura-Utsunomiya [3], Keiichi Hara [4], Miori Yuasa [5], Yuki Hasegawa [6], Hideo Sasai [7] and Satoshi Okada [2]

1. Division of Neonatal Screening, Research Institute, National Center for Child Health and Development, 2-10-1 Okura, Setagaya-ku, Tokyo 157-8535, Japan
2. Department of Pediatrics, Hiroshima University Graduate School of Biomedical and Health Sciences, 1-2-3 Kasumi, Minami-ku, Hiroshima 734-8551, Japan; rekagawa@hiroshima-u.ac.jp (R.K.); d185866@hiroshima-u.ac.jp (F.S.); sokada@hiroshima-u.ac.jp (S.O.)
3. Department of Pediatrics, Hiroshima Prefectural Hospital, 1-5-54 Ujinakanda, Minami-ku, Hiroshima 734-8530, Japan; a-utsunomiya@hph.pref.hiroshima.jp
4. Department of Pediatrics, National Hospital Organization Kure Medical Center and Chugoku Cancer Center, 3-1 Aoyama-cho, Kure 737-0023, Japan; hara.keiichi.dv@mail.hosp.go.jp
5. Department of Pediatrics, Faculty of Medical Sciences, University of Fukui, 23-3 Matsuoka-Shimoaizuki, Eiheiji-cho, Fukui 910-1193, Japan; miori@u-fukui.ac.jp
6. Department of Pediatrics, Japanese Red Cross Matsue Hospital, 200 Horomachi, Matsue 690-8506, Japan; yukirin@med.shimane-u.ac.jp
7. Department of Pediatrics, Graduate School of Medicine, Gifu University, 1-1 Yanagido, Gifu 501-1194, Japan; sasai@gifu-u.ac.jp
* Correspondence: tajima-g@ncchd.go.jp; Tel.: +81-3-5494-7133

Abstract: Propionic acidemia (PA) is a disorder of organic acid metabolism which typically presents with acute encephalopathy-like symptoms associated with metabolic acidosis and hyperammonemia during the neonatal period. The estimated incidence of symptomatic PA in Japan is 1/400,000. The introduction of neonatal screening using tandem mass spectrometry has revealed a far higher disease frequency of approximately 1/45,000 live births due to a prevalent variant of c.1304T>C (p.Y435C) in *PCCB*, which codes β-subunit of propionyl-CoA carboxylase. Our questionnaire-based follow-up study reveals that most of these patients remain asymptomatic. However, reports on symptomatic patients exhibiting cardiac complications such as cardiomyopathy and QT prolongation have been increasing. Moreover, there were even cases in which these cardiac complications were the only symptoms related to PA. A currently ongoing study is investigating the risk of cardiac complications in patients with neonatal screening-detected PA caused by this common variant.

Keywords: propionic acidemia; tandem mass spectrometry; propionylcarnitine; cardiomyopathy; QT prolongation

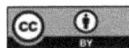

1. Introduction

Propionic acidemia (PA) is a disorder of organic acid metabolism that results from a congenital deficiency of propionyl-CoA carboxylase (PCC), which is composed of α- and β-subunits, which are coded by *PCCA* (MIM *232000, 13q32.3) and *PCCB* (MIM *232050, 3q22.3), respectively. PCC is located on the catabolic pathway of valine and isoleucine and catalyzes the conversion of propionyl-CoA to methylmalonyl-CoA in the mitochondrial matrix (Figure 1). Deficient PCC activity leads to the accumulation of toxic organic acids such as 3-hydroxypropionate and 2-methylcitrate. Typically, affected patients suffer from an acute acidotic crisis during the neonatal period and present with encephalopathy-like symptoms associated with metabolic acidosis and hyperammonemia immediately after the initiation of lactation, which often leaves neurological sequelae. Similarly, patients with milder phenotypes can show an acute disease onset in infancy or later. Various documented complications of PA include growth and psychomotor retardation, extrapyramidal disorder, cardiac disease, pancreatitis, hearing loss, and optic nerve atrophy. Prevention of disease progression in patients with PA requires a dietary restriction of precursor amino acids (i.e., valine, isoleucine, methionine, threonine, and glycine) accompanied with L-carnitine supplementation. Liver transplantation is considered in patients with poor disease control [1,2].

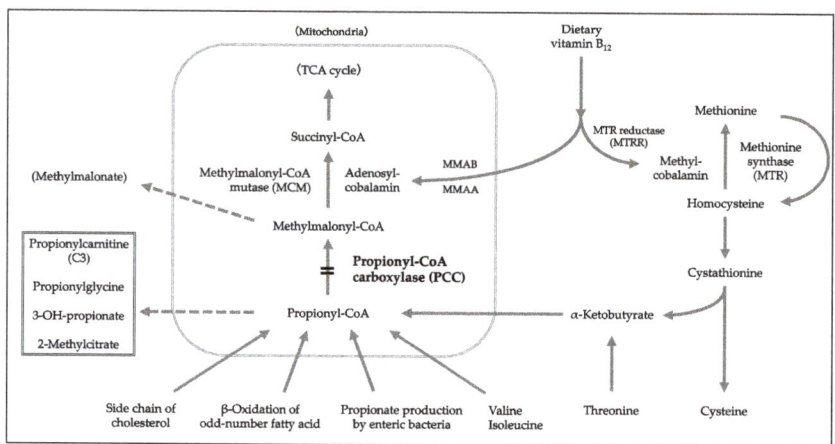

Figure 1. Metabolic pathways related to propionic acidemia. Dashed arrows are alternative pathways leading to disease-specific abnormal metabolites.

Aiming at improving the prognosis, several countries list PA as one of the target diseases for neonatal screening, but its utility is not established [1,3]. This review outlines the current perspectives on neonatal screening for PA in Japan.

2. Epidemiology in Japan

Before the introduction of neonatal screening using tandem mass spectrometry (MS/MS), the estimated incidence of patients with symptomatic PA was 1/400,000 in Japan. A study previously reported that c.923dupT, c.1196G>A (p.R399Q), and IVS18−6C>G in *PCCA* and c.1228C>T (p.R410W), c.1283C>T (p.T428I), and c.457>C (p.A153P) in *PCCB* were predominant genotypes in symptomatic Japanese patients with PA [4].

A pilot study on MS/MS-based neonatal screening was initiated in 1997 in several areas of the country, and 1,950,000 newborns, corresponding to approximately twice as many live births per year in Japan, were screened throughout the study period. Based on the results, the frequency of PA was 1/45,000, and the unexpectedly high detection rate was due to the presence of c.1304T>C (p.Y435C), a common variant of *PCCB*, with the estimated frequency of heterozygous carriers being 1/86.5 [5]. Homozygotes of the p.Y435C variant were proposed to be classified as those with mildest-type PA as it had not been detected in symptomatic patients.

3. Neonatal Screening for PA in Japan: Issues to Be Addressed

After the conclusion of the 15-year pilot study, MS/MS-based neonatal screening was adopted as an official public health service in 2013. The practice of neonatal screening is managed by 60 local public bodies, and the screening tests are assigned to 35 regional laboratories. Propionic acidemia has been included as one of the primary target diseases. Dried blood specimens are usually collected on the fourth or fifth day after birth, as has been done since the introduction of neonatal screening by the Guthrie method in 1977. Though earlier sample collection is thought to be more desirable for MS/MS-based neonatal screening and actually adopted in many countries [6], it has not been approved by the regulatory authority in Japan.

Under this condition, PA and methylmalonic acidemia (MMA) are screened using propionylcarnitine (C3) and the ratio of C3 to acetylcarnitine (C2) as indices. Cutoffs are generally set at 3.6 nmol/mL for C3 and 0.24 for C3/C2. Second-tier tests for C3 and C3/C2-positive dried blood specimens, measuring specific organic acids (3-hidroxypropionate, 2-methylcitrate, methylalonate) and total homocysteine by liquid chromatography-mass spectrometry, can be useful to improve sensitivity and specificity, but they are not available in most laboratories for the lack of official financial support, except in a few laboratories which have the budget for research purpose.

As confirmatory tests for positive subjects, the following biochemical analyses are recommended in the domestic guidelines edited by the Japanese Society for Inherited Metabolic Diseases (JSIMD): organic acids in urine, acylcarnitines, and vitamin B_{12} in serum, amino acids, and total homocysteine in plasma. Results of these biochemical tests are further confirmed by gene panel analysis including *PCCA*, *PCCB*, *MUT*, and genes in the pathway of adenosylcobalamin and methylcobalamin synthesis. Enzymatic assay of neither PCC nor methylmalonyl-CoA mutase (MCM) is supported by the national health insurance system, and they are offered by a few researchers.

Due to strict regulation by the Act on the Protection of Personal Information, it is quite difficult to collect data from each local public body and evaluate them centrally. Japanese Society for Neonatal Screening (JSNS) has collected statistical data on results of neonatal screening tests from each regional laboratory. During the period from 2015 to 2019, 4,715,965 newborns were screened, and the rates of dried blood specimen recollection and close examination for "C3 and C3/C2" were 0.059% and 0.006%, respectively. Though the data did not include detailed information on diagnostic findings of individual patients, positive predictive values for PA and MMA were 30.53% and 9.47%, respectively (partly available at https://www.jsms.gr.jp/contents03-05.html, written in Japanese, accessed on 18 June 2021).

The discrepancy between the frequency of symptomatic patients and that of patients detected by neonatal screening has illustrated that it is unclear what percentage of PA cases detected by neonatal screening is associated with the actual risk of clinical presentation. At the beginning of the pilot study on MS/MS-based neonatal screening, we expected to detect PA patients who were at the risk of presenting with acute metabolic decompensation and/or developing damage in central nervous system. The pilot study and the following official screening program revealed an unexpectedly high frequency of PA due to a common variant *PCCB* p.Y435C. However, it has been difficult to conclude them as false positive subjects, for PCC activities in their lymphocytes were reported to be as low as 3–8% of normal control value [5,7]. Therefore, it is important to determine newborns who will need medical management, which will also reduce the burden of unnecessary anxiety and treatment for patients who will remain asymptomatic throughout life [8]. Further scientific evidence is required to optimize neonatal screening for PA in Japan.

3.1. Correlation between Genotypes and Clinical/Biochemical Phenotypes

In 2015, we started a countrywide investigation by sending a preliminary questionnaire to 155 hospitals that were responsible for the management of neonatal screening-positive cases in Japan. Responses were collected from 130 hospitals (84%), and 87 patients with PA detected by neonatal screening, and 27 patients with symptomatic PA were identified. The summary of medical information of all 87 patients with neonatal screening-detected PA as well as 15 patients with symptomatic PA is shown in Table 1. Their diagnoses were confirmed by urinary organic acid analysis, using 3-hydroxypropionate, 2-methylcitrate, and propionylglycine as index metabolites. Some of the patients with neonatal screening-detected PA were as old as 20 years of age, and mental retardation was documented in one patient lacking any other PA-associated symptoms. The remaining patients were apparently healthy with no symptoms related to PA. Concerning biochemical examinations, a previous report suggested ketone bodies to be more useful for the evaluation of metabolic stability than the diagnostic metabolites [9]. In our study, mild elevation of total ketone bodies without symptoms was observed in regular examination of 7 neonatal screening-detected patients. Genetic analysis was performed in 72 patients, and the *PCCB* p.Y435C variant was detected in 61 patients, including 41 homozygotes, 16 compound heterozygotes with other *PCCB* variants, and 4 heterozygotes who were not checked for other variants. Six patients who were also checked only for the *PCCB* p.Y435C variant did not harbor it. Biallelic variants of *PCCA* were detected in 5 patients. There were no significant differences in the distributions of C3 and C3/C2 among these genotypes (Figure 2).

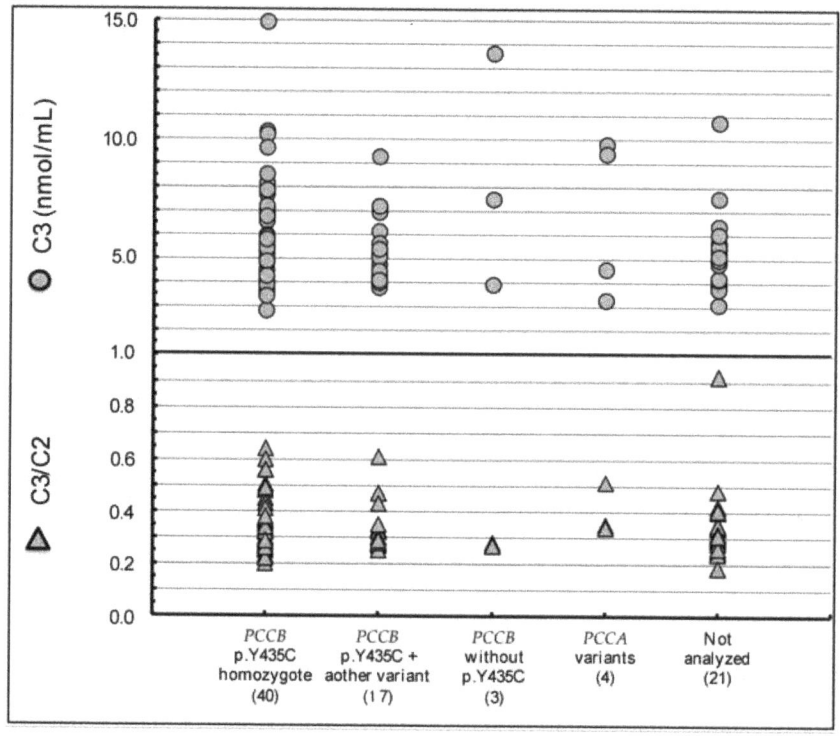

Figure 2. Distributions of propionylcarnitine (C3) and the ratio of C3 to acetylcarnitine (C2) in dried blood specimens of patients detected by neonatal screening. There are no significant differences among the genotypes.

Clinical disease onset manifested as acute acidotic crisis during the neonatal and infantile periods in 12 of the 15 patients with symptomatic PA. The remaining three patients had no history of acute metabolic failure, and clues to the diagnosis of PA were mental retardation in 2 patients and syncope in one patient who was subsequently diagnosed with QT prolongation. Genotypes were confirmed in 9 symptomatic patients. Biallelic *PCCB* variants were detected in 4 patients, none of whom harbored the p.Y435C variant. The remaining 5 patients had disease-causing *PCCA* variants.

Table 1. Clinical symptoms and genotypes of patients with propionic acidemia in Japan.

	Propionic Acidemia Detected by Neonatal Screening (n = 87)		Symptomatic Patients (n = 15)	
	Clinical phenotypes (n)			
	None	86	Acute acidotic crisis, neonatal onset	9
			Acute acidotic crisis, infantile onset	3
	Mental retardation	1	Mental retardation	2
			Syncope	1
	Genetic variants (n)			
PCCB	p.Y435C homozygote	41	p.T428I homozygote	1
	p.Y435C + p.T428I	5	p.T428I + frameshift variant	1
	p.Y435C + another variant	11	Other biallelic variants	2
	p.Y435C heterozygote [1]	4	p.Y435C detected	0
	p.Y435C not detected [1]	6		
PCCA	Biallelic variants detected	5	Biallelic variants detected	5
	No information of genotypes	15	No information of genotypes	6

[1] Variants other than PCCB p.Y435C were not analyzed.

Among the *PCCB* variants, c.1283C>T (p.T428I) was detected both in patients with neonatal screening-detected PA and in those with symptomatic PA. One patient with symptomatic PA who presented with an acute acidotic crisis during the neonatal period was confirmed to be homozygous for p.T428I, indicating that this variant caused a severe deficiency in PCC enzymatic activity. Five patients with neonatal screening-detected PA were compound heterozygotes for p.T428I and p.Y435C; all of them remained asymptomatic despite minimal medical management consisting of regular physical and biochemical examinations with or without L-carnitine supplementation. These findings suggest that patients with one p.Y435C allele should be expected to be free from the symptoms of PA.

In addition to the abovementioned questionnaire-based study, we have been prospectively collecting the genotypic information of neonatal screening target diseases, including PA, on a larger scale since 2014, based on gene panel analysis using next-generation sequencing with the MiSeq Sequencing System (Illumina, San Diego, CA, USA) performed at the Kazusa DNA Research Institute (Chiba, Japan). The details of the data on *PCCA* and *PCCB* variants are summarized in Table 2. In that cohort, among 58 patients with neonatal screening-detected PA, 31 (53%) were homozygous for p.Y435C, and 17 (29%) were compound heterozygotes for p.Y435C with another variant. In total, 48 of the 58 patients with neonatal screening-detected PA (83%) harbored p.Y435C in at least one allele. None of the 6 symptomatic patients harbored the p.Y435C variant.

Table 2. Frequencies of major variants in the larger-scale prospective study.

Patients	Gene and Variant	Allele Frequency
Patients detected by neonatal screening (n = 58)	PCCB p.Y435C	79/116 (68.1%)
	PCCB p.T428I	7/116 (6.0%)
	PCCB p.I430L	3/116 (2.6%)
	PCCB p.S510del	2/116 (1.7%)
Symptomatic patients (n = 6)	PCCA p.L308fs	2/11 (18.2%)
	PCCA p.W559L	2/11 (18.2%)

3.2. Potential Risk of Cardiac Complications in Asymptomatic Patients Detected by Neonatal Screening

Guidelines for the diagnosis and management of PA based on the clinical features of patients studied in large scales were published in 2014 [10] and revised in 2021 [1]. It has become clear that cardiac complications, mainly cardiomyopathy and QT prolongation, are quite specific to PA compared with other similar organic acid disorders and that these complications are primary causes of death during the chronic phase of PA [1,11–14]. Though precise pathophysiology has not been fully understood, mitochondrial impairment is suggested for the development of cardiomyopathy [2,15], and acute reduction of the repolarizing potassium currents in cardiomyocytes due to toxic metabolites for the prolonged QTc interval [2,16].

In the present study, cardiomyopathy and/or QT prolongation was observed in 6 out of the 15 symptomatic patients (Table 3). Four of these patients with cardiac complications suffered an acute acidotic crisis, whereas the remaining 2 patients did not have a history of acute metabolic failure, indicating that cardiac lesions could develop regardless of the severity of metabolic derangement, as was suggested in previous reports [12,14,17,18].

Table 3. Cardiac complications observed in symptomatic patients.

Clinical Phenotype	Number of Patients	Cardiac Complication	Cardiac Findings
Acute acidotic crisis, neonatal onset	9	3	Cardiomyopathy + ventricular tachycardia
			Left ventricular dilatation + QT prolongation
			Mild tricuspid regurgitation
Acute acidotic crisis, infantile onset	3	2	Left ventricular dilatation + mild mitral regurgitation
			QT prolongation
Chronic symptoms only	3	2	QT prolongation
			QT prolongation with syncope
Total	15	7	

These findings raise the question of whether apparently healthy patients with neonatal screening-detected PA in Japan can also develop similar cardiac complications. As an additional study started in 2017, we collected data on cardiac ultrasonography and electrocardiography from 45 and 50 patients, respectively, within the cohort of 87 patients with neonatal screening-detected PA. We did not observe abnormalities except cardiomyopathic changes in one patient, whose genotype has not yet been determined. Thus far, cardiac complications have not been reported in any of the patients who are homozygous for p.Y435C. However, it may require the observation of one generation to clarify whether these patients with mildest-type PA may also develop cardiac lesions in a prospective cohort follow-up study.

To address this uncertainty in a shorter time period, we have planned to search for patients with occult PA by measuring 3-hydroxypropionate and 2-methylcitrate levels in urine and C3 levels in serum in patients with cardiomyopathy and/or QT prolongation. Those with abnormal results will be further analyzed for genotyping. Patients with PA detected in this study may benefit from nutritional therapy and L-carnitine supplementation to reduce the accumulation of abnormal metabolites, though the effects of these therapies on the cardiac complications are not proven [1]. Romano et al. reported that liver transplantation improved not only acidotic symptoms but also cardiomyopathy in patients with PA [12]. In the latest guidelines, however, the recommendation of liver transplantation for PA-based cardiomyopathy is still withheld because there have been unfavorable reports on cases that developed cardiomyopathy after liver transplantation as well as reports on successful cases [1].

4. Conclusions

Currently implemented neonatal screening for PA in Japan unexpectedly has led to the detection of a high frequency of patients with PA. Most of these patients detected by neonatal screening harbor at least one *PCCB* p.Y435C allele, which appears to retain sufficient enzymatic function to prevent clinical disease onset. Neonatal screening should not burden newborns and their parents with unnecessary anxiety by overdiagnosis or unnecessary treatment; therefore, the clinical significance of this genotype must be clarified.

Author Contributions: Project administration and original draft preparation, G.T.; questionnaire studies, R.K., F.S., A.N.-U., K.H., M.Y., Y.H.; prospective collection of genotypic information and funding acquisition, H.S.; supervision, S.O. All authors have read and agreed to the published version of the manuscript.

Funding: This work was partly supported by Japan Agency for Medical Research and Development (AMED) under Grant Numbers (1) JP16ek0109050, JP19ek0109276, Chief Investigator: Toshiyuki Fukao, and (2) JP21ek0109482, Chief Investigator: Hideo Sasai.

Institutional Review Board Statement: The study was conducted according to the guidelines of the Declaration of Helsinki, and approved by the Ethics Committee of National Center for Child Health and Development (protocol No.1250, approved on 18 August 2016 and 27 March 2018; No. 1529, 22 August 2017; No. 1547, 22 August 2017; No. 2020-233, 8 December 2020).

Informed Consent Statement: Informed consent was obtained from all subjects involved in the study.

Data Availability Statement: The data presented in this study are available on request from the corresponding author.

Acknowledgments: The authors thank Haruko Kitazawa and Akiko Shimura, Division of Neonatal Screening, Research Institute, National Center for Child Health and Development, for their support in conducting the questionnaire studies.

Conflicts of Interest: The authors declare no conflict of interest.

References

1. Forny, P.; Höster, F.; Ballhausen, D.; Chakrapani, A.; Chapman, K.A.; Dionisi-Vici, C.; Dixon, M.; Grünert, S.C.; Grunewald, S.; Haliloglu, G.; et al. Guidelines for the diagnosis and management of methylmalonic acidaemia and propionic acidaemia: First revision. *J. Inherit. Metab. Dis.* **2021**, *44*, 566–592. [CrossRef] [PubMed]
2. Haijes, H.A.; Jans, J.J.M.; Tas, S.Y.; Verhoeven-Duif, N.M.; van Hasselt, P.M. Pathophysiology of propionic and methylmalonic acidemias. Part 1: Complications. *J. Inherit. Metab. Dis.* **2019**, *42*, 730–744. [CrossRef] [PubMed]
3. Haijes, H.A.; van Hasselt, P.M.; Jans, J.J.M.; Tas, S.Y.; Verhoeven-Duif, N.M. Pathophysiology of propionic and methylmalonic acidemias. Part 2: Treatment strategies. *J. Inherit. Metab. Dis.* **2019**, *42*, 745–761. [CrossRef] [PubMed]
4. Yang, X.; Sakamoto, O.; Matsubara, Y.; Kure, S.; Suzuki, Y.; Aoki, Y.; Yamaguchi, S.; Takahashi, Y.; Nishikubo, T.; Kawaguchi, C.; et al. Mutation spectrum of the *PCCA* and *PCCB* genes in Japanese patients with propionic acidemia. *Mol. Genet. Metab.* **2004**, *81*, 335–342. [CrossRef] [PubMed]
5. Yorifuji, T.; Kawai, M.; Muroi, J.; Mamada, M.; Kurokawa, K.; Shigematsu, Y.; Hirano, S.; Sakura, N.; Yoshida, I.; Kuhara, T.; et al. Unexpectedly high prevalence of the mild form of propionic acidemia in Japan: Presence of a common mutation and possible clinical implications. *Hum. Genet.* **2002**, *111*, 161–165. [CrossRef] [PubMed]
6. Heringer, J.; Valayannopoulos, V.; Lund, A.M.; Wijburg, F.A.; Freisinger, P.; Barić, I.; Baumgartner, M.R.; Burgard, P.; Burlina, A.B.; Chapman, K.A.; et al. Impact of age at onset and newborn screening on outcome in organic acidurias. *J. Inherit. Metab. Dis.* **2016**, *39*, 341–353. [CrossRef] [PubMed]
7. Gotoh, K.; Nakajima, Y.; Tajima, G.; Watanabe, Y.; Hotta, Y.; Kataoka, T.; Kawade, Y.; Sugiyama, N.; Ito, T.; Kimura, K.; et al. Determination of methylmalonyl coenzyme A by ultra high-performance liquid chromatography tandem mass spectrometry for measuring propionyl coenzyme A carboxylase activity in patients with propionic acidemia. *J. Chromatogr. B Anal. Technol. Biomed. Life Sci.* **2017**, *1046*, 195–199. [CrossRef] [PubMed]
8. Haijes, H.A.; Molema, F.; Langeveld, M.; Janssen, M.C.; Bosch, A.M.; van Spronsen, F.; Mulder, M.F.; Verhoeven-Duif, N.M.; Jans, J.J.M.; van der Ploeg, A.T.; et al. Retrospective evaluation of the Dutch pre-newborn screening cohort for propionic acidemia and isolated methylmalonic acidemia: What to aim, expect, and evaluate from newborn screening? *J. Inherit. Metab. Dis.* **2020**, *43*, 424–437. [CrossRef] [PubMed]

9. Haijes, H.S.; Jans, J.J.M.; van der Ham, M.; van Hasselt, P.M.; Verhoeven-Duif, N.M. Understanding acute metabolic decompensateion in propionic and methylalonic acidemias: A deep metabolic phenotyping approach. *Orphanet J. Rare Dis.* **2020**, *15*, 68. [CrossRef] [PubMed]
10. Baumgartner, M.R.; Hörster, F.; Dionisi-Vici, C.; Haliloglu, G.; Karall, D.; Chapman, K.A.; Huemer, M.; Hochuli, M.; Assoun, M.; Ballhausen, D.; et al. Proposed guidelines for the diagnosis and management of methylmalonic and propionic acidemia. *Orphanet J. Rare Dis.* **2014**, *9*, 130–165. [CrossRef] [PubMed]
11. Pena, L.; Burton, B.K. Survey of health status and complications among propionic acidemia patients. *Am. J. Med. Genet. A* **2012**, *158A*, 1641–1646. [CrossRef] [PubMed]
12. Romano, S.; Valayannopoulos, V.; Touati, G.; Jais, J.P.; Rabier, D.; de Keyzer, Y.; Bonnet, D.; de Lonlay, P. Cardiomyopathies in propionic aciduria are reversible after liver transplantation. *J. Pediatr.* **2010**, *156*, 128–134. [CrossRef] [PubMed]
13. Kölker, S.; Valayannopoulos, V.; Burlina, A.B.; Sykut-Cegielska, J.; Wijburg, F.A.; Teles, E.L.; Zeman, J.; Dionisi-Vici, C.; Barić, I.; Karall, D.; et al. The phenotypic spectrum of organic acidurias and urea cycle disorders. Part 2. The evolving clinical phenotype. *J. Inherit. Metab. Dis.* **2015**, *38*, 1059–1074. [CrossRef] [PubMed]
14. Baumgartner, D.; Scholl-Bürgi, S.; Sass, J.O.; Sperl, W.; Schweigmann, U.; Stein, J.I.; Karall, D. Prolonged QTc intervals and decreased left ventricular contractility in patients with propionic acidemia. *J. Pediatr.* **2007**, *150*, 192–197. [CrossRef] [PubMed]
15. Baruteau, J.; Hargreaves, I.; Krywawych, S.; Chalasani, A.; Land, J.M.; Davison, J.E.; Kwok, M.K.; Christov, G.; Karimova, A.; Ashworth, M.; et al. Successful reversal of propionic acidaemia associated cardiomyopathy: Evidence for low myocardial coenzyme Q10 status and secondary mitochondrial dysfunction as an underlying pathophysiological mechanism. *Mitochondrion* **2014**, *17*, 150–156. [CrossRef] [PubMed]
16. Bodi, I.; Grünert, S.C.; Becker, N.; Stoelzle-Feix, S.; Spiekerkoetter, U.; Zehender, M.; Bugger, H.; Bode, C.; Odening, K.E. Mechanisms of acquired long QT syndrome in patients with propionic academia. *Heart Rhythm* **2016**, *13*, 1335–1345. [CrossRef] [PubMed]
17. Riemersma, M.; Hazebroek, M.R.; Helderman-van den Enden, A.T.J.M.; Salomons, G.S.; Ferdinandusse, S.; Brouwers, M.C.G.; van der Ploeg, L.; Heymans, S.; Glatz, J.F.C.; van den Wijngaard, A.; et al. Propionic acidemia as a cause of adult-onset dilated cardiomyopathy. *Eur. J. Hum. Genet.* **2017**, *25*, 1195–1201. [CrossRef] [PubMed]
18. Kölker, S.; Cazorla, A.G.; Valayannopoulos, V.; Lund, A.M.; Burlina, A.B.; Sykut-Cegielska, J.; Wijburg, F.A.; Teles, E.L.; Zeman, J.; Dionisi-Vici, C.; et al. The phenotypic spectrum of organic acidurias and urea cycle disorders. Part 1: The initial presentation. *J. Inherit. Metab. Dis.* **2015**, *38*, 1041–1057. [CrossRef]

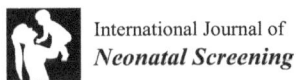

Article

Pilot Study on Neonatal Screening for Methylmalonic Acidemia Caused by Defects in the Adenosylcobalamin Synthesis Pathway and Homocystinuria Caused by Defects in Homocysteine Remethylation

Reiko Kagawa [1], Go Tajima [1,2,*], Takako Maeda [2], Fumiaki Sakura [1], Akari Nakamura-Utsunomiya [3], Keiichi Hara [4], Yutaka Nishimura [5], Miori Yuasa [6], Yosuke Shigematsu [6], Hiromi Tanaka [7], Saki Fujihara [7], Chiyoko Yoshii [7] and Satoshi Okada [1]

1. Department of Pediatrics, Hiroshima University Graduate School of Biomedical and Health Sciences, Minami-ku, Hiroshima 734-8551, Japan; rekagawa@hiroshima-u.ac.jp (R.K.); d185866@hiroshima-u.ac.jp (F.S.); sokada@hiroshima-u.ac.jp (S.O.)
2. Division of Neonatal Screening, Research Institute, National Center for Child Health and Development, Setagaya-ku, Tokyo 157-8535, Japan; maeda-t@ncchd.go.jp
3. Department of Pediatrics, Hiroshima Prefectural Hospital, Minami-ku, Hiroshima 734-8530, Japan; a-utsunomiya@hph.pref.hiroshima.jp
4. Department of Pediatrics, National Hospital Organization Kure Medical Center and Chugoku Cancete Center, Kure 737-0023, Japan; hara.keiichi.dv@mail.hosp.go.jp
5. Department of General Perinatology, Hiroshima City Hiroshima Citizens Hospital, Naka-Ku, Hiroshima 730-8518, Japan; warabikinako@gmail.com
6. Department of Pediatrics, Faculty of Medical Sciences, University of Fukui, Eiheiji-cho, Fukui 910-1193, Japan; miori@u-fukui.ac.jp (M.Y.); yosuke@u-fukui.ac.jp (Y.S.)
7. Hiroshima City Medical Association Clinical Laboratory, Naka-ku, Hiroshima 730-8611, Japan; saiboushin@labo.city.hiroshima.med.or.jp (H.T.); sententaisha@labo.city.hiroshima.med.or.jp (S.F.); yoshii@labo.city.hiroshima.med.or.jp (C.Y.)
* Correspondence: tajima-g@ncchd.go.jp; Tel.: +81-3-5494-7133

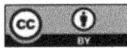

Abstract: Neonatal screening (NS) for methylmalonic acidemia uses propionylcarnitine (C3) as a primary index, which is insufficiently sensitive at detecting methylmalonic acidemia caused by defects in the adenosylcobalamin synthesis pathway. Moreover, homocystinuria from cystathionine β-synthase deficiency is screened by detecting hypermethioninemia, but methionine levels decrease in homocystinuria caused by defects in homocysteine remethylation. To establish NS detection of methylmalonic acidemia and homocystinuria of these subtypes, we evaluated the utility of indices (1) C3 $\geq$ 3.6 µmol/L and C3/acetylcarnitine (C2) $\geq$ 0.23, (2) C3/methionine $\geq$ 0.25, and (3) methionine < 10 µmol/L, by retrospectively applying them to NS data of 59,207 newborns. We found positive results in 116 subjects for index (1), 37 for (2), and 15 for (3). Second-tier tests revealed that for index 1, methylmalonate (MMA) was elevated in two cases, and MMA and total homocysteine (tHcy) were elevated in two cases; for index 2 that MMA was elevated in one case; and for index 3 that tHcy was elevated in one case. Though data were anonymized, two cases identified by index 1 had been diagnosed with maternal vitamin B_{12} deficiency during NS. Methylene tetrahydrofolate reductase deficiency was confirmed for the case identified by index 3, which was examined because an elder sibling was affected by the same disease. Based on these data, a prospective NS study is underway.

Keywords: neonatal screening; homocystinuria; methylmalonic acidemia; disorders of cobalamin metabolism; hypomethioninemia

1. Introduction

Current neonatal screening (NS) in Japan identifies methylmalonic acidemia and propionic acidemia by elevated levels of propionylcarnitine (C3), and homocystinuria caused from cystathionine β-synthase (CBS) deficiency by elevated levels of methionine (Met). However, C3 is not always sufficiently sensitive to detect methylmalonic acidemia caused by defects in the adenosylcobalamin synthesis pathway, as we show below in a case of cobalamin D disease (cblD) variant 2 missed in NS. Moreover, Met levels actually decrease in homocystinuria resulting from defects in homocysteine remethylation. The prognosis of these diseases can be greatly improved by starting specific medication in the early neonatal period [1–7], as observed through the management of two siblings affected by methylenetetrahydrofolate reductase (MTHFR) deficiency, which is described below.

2. Materials and Methods

2.1. Preliminary Retrospective Study

In Japan, dried blood spot (DBS) testing for NS generally takes place on the fourth or fifth day after birth. In the Hiroshima area, there are approximately 20,000 births each year, and all NS samples are analyzed in the Hiroshima City Medical Association Clinical Laboratory. To improve the sensitivity of current NS for methylmalonic acidemia caused by defects in the adenosylcobalamin synthesis pathway and to establish NS for homocystinuria caused by defects in homocysteine remethylation, we planned a preliminary retrospective study to apply the following indices to NS data from April 2015 to September 2017: (1) C3 and C3/acetylcarnitine (C2) (current NS indices for methylmalonic acidemia and propionic acidemia), (2) C3/Met, and (3) Met (the lower cutoff).

2.2. Prospective Pilot Study

After evaluating positive rates for each index, we enrolled newborns from 10 major hospitals in the Hiroshima area into a pilot study on prospective NS. Parents provided their written informed consent for participation. Samples were anonymized by the removal of personal information. Samples that met one or more of the three indices were transported to the National Center for Child Health and Development for the second-tier measurement of methylmalonate (MMA) and total homocysteine (tHcy). Patients with elevated MMA and/or tHcy were further examined in the Department of Pediatrics, Hiroshima University Hospital.

2.3. Biochemical Analysis

Analysis of amino acids and acylcarnitines in the NS DBS was performed using the flow injection method with an LCMS-8030 tandem mass spectrometer (Shimadzu, Kyoto, Japan). The second-tier measurement of MMA and tHcy in DBS was performed using liquid chromatography–mass spectrometry with an LCMS-8040 tandem mass spectrometer (Shimadzu). Cutoff values for MMA and tHcy were 1 µmol/L and 5 µmol/L, respectively.

2.4. Statistical Analysis

Statistical analyses of NS test results were performed using a Tandem Internal Quality Control System (System Kay, Kyoto, Japan) and Histogram Creation Sheet (Technical Subcommittee, Japanese Society for Neonatal Screening, Tokyo, Japan).

3. Case Report

3.1. Case 1

A baby boy born as the first child of healthy nonconsanguineous parents at 37 weeks' gestation weighed 2864 g at birth. His NS DBS showed that C3 level was elevated to 4.79 nmol/mL (cutoff, 3.6 nmol/mL), but C3/C2 was considered normal at 0.231 (cutoff, 0.25). He showed normal growth and psychomotor development. At 1 year of age, he had norovirus gastroenteritis, presenting with vomiting, groaning, and impaired consciousness, and was taken to an emergency hospital. Blood tests revealed marked acidosis, and plasma ammonia was elevated to 251 µg/dL (normal range, 30–80 µg/dL). Further diagnostic analysis revealed plasma MMA levels of 132.7 nmol/mL (normal range, 0.23–0.45 nmol/mL), suggestive of MMA. Lymphocyte methylmalonyl-CoA mutase activity was normal in the presence of adenosylcobalamin (56.2 pmol succinyl-CoA/min/ 10^6 cells, control 61.6 ± 22.2). His serum tHcy and vitamin B_{12} levels were normal. Based on these results, he was diagnosed with suspected vitamin B_{12}-responsive methylmalonic acidemia. A vitamin B_{12} challenge test was performed by daily infusion of 1 mg cyanocobalamin for 5 days. Post-challenge, his MMA levels decreased. Genetic analysis revealed compound heterozygous variants in *MMADHC*; c.18T > A (p.C6X) and c.702insT. Based on a diagnosis of CblD (variant 2), cobalamin and carnitine therapy was started. This case was reported previously [8].

3.2. Case 2

A baby girl born as the first child of healthy nonconsanguineous parents at 40 weeks' gestation weighed 2810 g at birth, and NS results were normal. However, her sucking was weak and her weight gain was poor. From 2.5 months of age, she presented with hypertonia and the setting-sun eye phenomenon. Although ultrasonography of her brain at 13 days old showed no abnormal findings (Figure 1), head magnetic resonance imaging (MRI) at 2.5 months revealed marked ventricular enlargement, suggesting hydrocephalus or brain atrophy (Figure 2). She underwent ventricular drainage, but respiratory failure became evident at 4 months of age when there was no improvement in head MRI findings. Further diagnostic analysis revealed plasma tHcy levels of 170 µmol/L (normal range, 3.7–13.5 µmol/L) and urinary Hcy levels of 510 µmol/mg·cre (reference value, "undetectable"), suggestive of homocystinuria. As plasma Met level was as low as 3.4 µmol/L (normal range, 18.9–40.5 µmol/L), defects in homocysteine remethylation were indicated. A Met decrease in the NS DBS was also ascertained retrospectively (6.6 µmol/L).

The administration of betaine monohydrate (100 mg/kg/day) was started at 4 months of age, and her respiratory status and vitality improved rapidly. Sanger sequencing of the methylenetetrahydrofolate reductase gene (*MTHFR*) detected a homozygous variant, c.466_467GC > TT, and both parents were found to be heterozygous carriers of this variant. Based on the diagnosis of homocystinuria type III caused by MTHFR deficiency, betaine therapy was continued at the dosage of 300 mg/kg/day, which raised plasma Met levels to 14–40 µmol/L, and reduced plasma tHcy concentrations to 50–110 µmol/L. Head MRI at the age of 12 months revealed the almost complete resolution of ventricular enlargement and atrophic changes (Figure 3). However, severe psychomotor retardation became evident, with a development quotient of 36 at the age of 1 year and 4 months. Epileptic seizures also appeared at the age of 3 years, so the administration of sodium valproate was added. This case was reported previously [9].

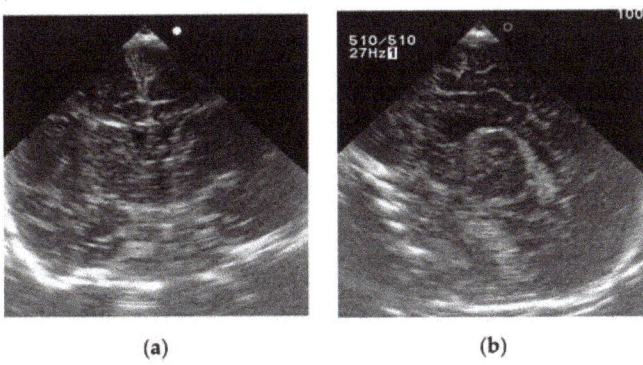

Figure 1. Brain ultrasonography of Case 2 at 13 days of age. (**a**) Coronal plane; (**b**) sagittal plane.

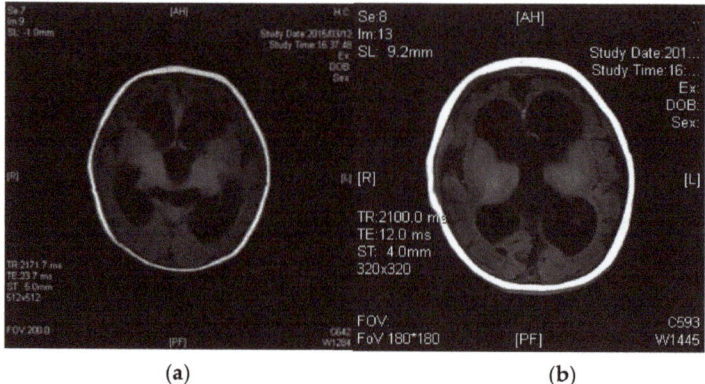

Figure 2. Brain MRI of Case 2. (**a**) At 2.5 months of age (T1); (**b**) 4 months of age (T1) showing no effect on the ventricular size after ventricular drainage.

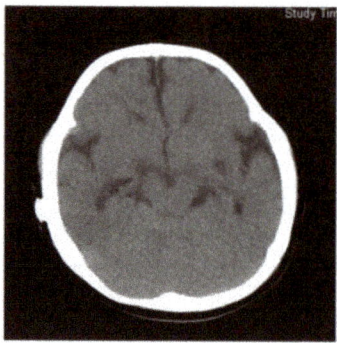

Figure 3. Brain CT of Case 2 at 12 months of age, 7 months after starting betaine treatment.

3.3. Case 3

A baby boy born as the second child of the same parents as Case 2 at the gestational age of 38 weeks and 5 days, with a birth weight of 2936 g, had a normal perinatal course. Due to the medical history of his sister (Case 2), blood samples were collected within 24 h of birth. Concentrations of Met in his DBS and plasma were 8.7 µmol/L and 5.4 µmol/L, respectively. Plasma tHcy levels were elevated to 97.4 µmol/L, which was associated with increased urinary Hcy levels (3437.1 µmol/mg·cre). These data suggested MTHFR deficiency, so the administration of betaine at 300 mg/day (approximately 100 mg/kg/day) was started at the age of 7 days. Thereafter, plasma Met and tHcy were controlled within the range of 12–15 µmol/L and 80–120 µmol/L, respectively. He has maintained normal growth and psychomotor development up to the age of 12 months, and no abnormalities were found on head MRI. This case was reported previously [9].

4. Results

4.1. Preliminary Retrospective Study

Prior to the preliminary retrospective study, we evaluated statistical data for C3, C3/C2, Met, and C3/Met in the DBS of 23,467 newborns in the Hiroshima area from April 2016 to March 2017 (Tables 1 and 2). The C3 cutoff has remained at 3.6 µmol/L since the start of tandem mass spectrometry (MS/MS)-based NS in 2013. This value corresponds to the 98.1st percentile of the enrolled data, resulting in a positive rate of 1.82%. The C3/C2 cutoff needs adjusting every few years, so was set at 0.22. The combination of cutoffs for C3 and C3/C2 yielded a positive rate of 0.09%. The 99.9th percentile and 99.5th percentile of C3/Met were 0.25 and 0.20, respectively. Setting the C3/Met cutoff at 0.25 (the 99.9th percentile) gave a positive rate of 0.13%, which was appropriate for the first screening test. However, a lower Met cutoff was required to detect MTHFR deficiency. Cutoffs of 9.0 µmol/L and 10.0 µmol/L achieved positive rates of 0.05% and 0.12%, respectively. Based on these data, we established the following cutoffs for the preliminary study: (1) C3 ≥ 3.6 µmol/L and C3/C2 ≥ 0.22, (2) C3/Met ≥ 0.25, and (3) Met < 10.0 µmol/L.

Table 1. Index distributions of dried blood spots from newborns in the Hiroshima area from April 2016 to March 2017 (n = 23,467).

	Mean	99th Centile	99.5th Centile	99.9th Centile
C3 (µmol/L)	1.83	3.96	4.36	5.8
C3/C2	0.09	0.18	0.19	0.24
C3/Met	0.08	0.18	0.20	0.25
Met (µmol/L)	22.10	34.71	36.60	41.75

Table 2. Newborns meeting different cutoff levels in the Hiroshima area from April 2016 to March 2017 (n = 23,437).

Index	Cutoff Level					
C3 (µmol/L)	3.5		3.6		3.7	
	n	%	n	%	n	%
	513	2.19	423	1.82	350	1.49
C3/C2 [1]	0.22		0.23		0.24	
	n	%	n	%	n	%
	30	0.12	23	0.09	15	0.06
C3/C2 and C3 ≥ 3.6 µmol/L [1]	0.22		0.23		0.24	
	n	%	n	%	n	%
	22	0.09	16	0.08	13	0.05
C3/Met [2]	0.24		0.25		0.26	
	n	%	n	%	n	%
	12	0.13	10	0.13	8	0.10
Met (µmol/L)	9		10		11	
	n	%	n	%	n	%
	11	0.05	28	0.12	56	0.24

[1] Data of 23,390 newborns; [2] data of 7714 newborns.

For the preliminary study, NS data of 59,207 newborns were evaluated, and a total of 116, 37, and 15 newborns were selected for second-tier tests using indices 1–3, respectively. For index 1, we observed a MMA increase in two cases, and increased MMA and tHcy in two cases. For index 2, we observed a MMA increase in one case. For index 3, we observed a tHcy increase in one case (Table 3). Though further examination was not included in this study, three out of the four cases assessed using index 1 were shown to be positive for screening with C3 and C3/C2 indicators in the current NS, and maternal vitamin B_{12} deficiency was confirmed in two of them. One case with increased MMA had no apparent cause. The case with increased tHcy measured using index 3 was Case 3 described above.

Table 3. Retrospective screening for disorders of cobalamin metabolism in 59,207 newborns in the Hiroshima area from April 2015 to September 2017.

Index	First Test (n)	Second-Tier Test (n)			
		Elevated MMA	Elevated MMA and tHcy	Elevated tHcy	Total
(1) C3 ≥ 3.6 μmol/L and C3/C2 ≥ 0.22	116	2	2	0	4
(2) C3/Met > 0.25 and Met < 10 μmol/L	37	1	0	0	1
(3) Met < 10 μmol/L	15	0	0	1	1
Total	168 (0.35%)	3	2	1	6 (3.67%)

Reference range: methylmalonate (MMA) < 1 μmol/L; total homocysteine (tHcy) < 5 μmol/L.

4.2. Prospective Pilot Study

Between April 2019 and December 2020, 6080 of 40,595 newborns in the Hiroshima area were enrolled in the pilot study. The C3/C2 cutoff is reviewed every few years, and was set at 0.23 from April 2019 (data not shown). Therefore, we set the C3/C2 cutoff to 0.23 in the prospective pilot study. The number of cases shown to be positive was two using index 1 alone, one using both indices 1 and 2, seven using index 2 alone, eight using indices 2 and 3, and 54 using index 3 alone (Table 4). Only one subject out of a total of 72 with a positive finding had increased MMA levels in the second-tier tests, but no increase in serum MMA or plasma tHcy was observed on detailed examination (data not shown). Additionally, no obvious pathological variants were detected in genes associated with cobalamin metabolism (*MMAA, MMAB, MMACHC, MMADHC*), *MUT*, *PCCA*, or *PCCB* (data not shown).

Table 4. Prospective pilot screening in the Hiroshima area from April 2019 to March 2021.

	Newborns Enrolled in This Study (n = 6080)	All Newborns in the Area (n = 40,595)
Index	First Test, n (%)	
(1) C3 ≥ 3.6 μmol/L and C3/C2 ≥ 0.23	3 (0.05)	21 *[1] (0.05)
(2) C3/Met > 0.25	15 *[2] (0.24)	54 *[3] (0.13)
(3) Met < 10 μmol/L	54 (0.89)	271 (0.05)
Total	72 (1.18)	346 (0.85)
	Second test, n	
Elevated MMA	1	ND
Elevated tHcy	0	ND

Reference range: methylmalonate (MMA) < 1 μmol/L; total homocysteine (tHcy) < 5 μmol/L. *[1] 4 using indices (1) and (2); *[2] 8 using indices (2) and (3); *[3] 10 using indices (2) and (3).

To investigate the low Met levels of low birth weight infants, each index was examined in the NS carried out from April to October 2019 for infants with a birth weight of ≤2000 g who were part of the pilot study. No association with low birth weight infants was found for index 1, but the frequency of low birth weight infants increased for indices 2 and 3 (Table 5).

Table 5. Correlation between low birth weight and hypomethioninemia.

	Birth Weight ≥ 2000 g, n (%)	Birth Weight < 2000 g, n (%)	p-Value
n (%)	12,191 (98.32)	209 (1.68)	
(1) C3 ≥ 3.6 µmol/L and C3/C2 ≥ 0.23	5 *[1] (0.04)	(0)	–
(2) C3/Met > 0.25	3 (0.02)	3 (1.43)	<0.001
(3) Met < 10 µmol/L	74 (0.61)	26 (12.44)	<0.001

*[1] 1 using indices (1) and (2).

5. Discussion

Fifteen years after the pilot study in 1997, MS/MS-based NS was adopted as an official Japanese public health care service in 2013 [11]. Its target diseases include methylmalonic acidemia and homocystinuria caused by CBS deficiency. In clinical practice, however, we encountered two symptomatic infants with biochemical profiles identical to those of methylmalonic acidemia who were diagnosed with cblD variant 2 (Case 1) and maternal vitamin B_{12} deficiency (data not shown), respectively, and their NS results were within normal range. Retrospective evaluation of NS data from the cblD patient revealed mild elevation of C3 with a C3/C2 value slightly below the cutoff. The first NS test for both C3 and C3/C2 had been positive in the patient with maternal vitamin B_{12} deficiency, but their second NS test was normal. Additionally, several previous studies reported that methylmalonic acidemia caused by defects in the adenosylcobalamin synthesis pathway tend to show only a slight increase in C3, if any, in neonatal DBS [1,2,11–13]. As the symptoms of some of these patients can easily be prevented by the specific administration of vitamin B_{12}, more sensitive NS tests are required to enable medication to be administered before the clinical onset of disease [1–3,11–14].

In the present study, we document our experience of two siblings with MTHFR deficiency who followed contrasting clinical courses. The differences in their prognoses appear to be dependent upon the timing when betaine therapy was started. Betaine (N,N,N-trimethylglycine) is the substrate for betaine-homocysteine methyltransferase (BHMT) and thus serves as a methyl donor instead of methylcobalamin. Though the physiological function of BHMT cannot compensate for methionine synthase which requires methylcobalamin, the pharmacological dosage of betaine is effective in reducing tHcy and increasing Met levels in the blood. Met is converted into S-adenosylmethionine (SAM), which is an important methyl donor for various methylation reactions. Therefore, maintaining normal levels of plasma Met is essential in preventing SAM deficiency, which causes severe damage to the central nervous system, especially during infancy and childhood. As it has been shown that the early introduction of betaine therapy can suppress the symptoms of homocystinuria caused by remethylation defects [1–7], a highly preventive effect of NS is expected. In our preliminary retrospective study, the Met cutoffs of 9.0 µmol/L and 10.0 µmol/L achieved positive rates of 0.05% and 0.12%, respectively, and none of the newborns had Met levels below 8.0 µmol/L. Referring to the cases of MTHFR deficiency that we experienced (Case 2) and previously reported cases, we set the Met cutoff at 10 µmol/L to perform more sensitive NS.

Several studies have been conducted on primary indices and second-tier tests to determine if they have sufficient sensitivity and specificity for screening for cobalamin metabolic disorders [2,10,12,13,15–17]. MMA and tHcy in DBS are recommended as promising metabolites for the second-tier measurement [1,2], but current NS practice for these diseases varies between countries [2]. In Japan, our pilot study is the first known trial of prospective screening. In the prospective pilot study, using indices C3, C3/C2, C3/Met, and Met with a lower cutoff increased the number of newborn babies targeted for the second-tier test to 1.18% (72 out of 6080 newborns). By combining the measurement of MMA and tHcy as a second-tier test, only one newborn was found to have an elevated

MMA level. Measuring MMA and tHcy as a second-tier is apparently useful in reducing false positives.

Our prospective pilot study raises the question of why the number of newborns with C3/Met levels above the cutoff and below the Met level were higher in the Hiroshima area during the study period. Taking into consideration the fact that newborns enrolled in this study were limited to those born in 10 major hospitals, of which many have a neonatal intensive care unit, and that the ratio of newborns enrolled in this study was as low as 15%, we speculate that the study group has a higher frequency of low birth weight infants than the surrounding area. Low birth weight and preterm infants were previously reported to have low levels of Met concentration in their blood [2], and our NS data suggest similar tendencies (Table 5).

6. Conclusions

Although no affected patients has been detected in our prospective pilot study so far, the use of indices C3, C3/C2, C3/Met, and Met with a lower cutoff in combination with second-tier measurements of MMA and tHcy seem to be promising in the establishment of NS for methylmalonic acidemia caused by defects in the adenosylcobalamin synthesis pathway and homocystinuria caused by defects in homocysteine remethylation. We should discuss in this study whether newborns with the real target disease can be detected, and if there are any undetected cases. The progress of future research will be clarified.

Author Contributions: Conceptualization, G.T.; methodology, G.T.; software, C.Y.; validation, R.K., C.Y. and G.T.; formal analysis, R.K. and C.Y.; investigation, R.K., T.M., H.T., S.F., C.Y., M.Y. and Y.S.; resources, R.K., F.S., A.N.-U., K.H. and Y.N.; data curation, R.K., G.T. and C.Y.; writing—original draft preparation, R.K.; writing—review and editing, G.T.; visualization, R.K., C.Y. and G.T.; supervision, G.T.; project administration, S.O.; funding acquisition, G.T. All authors have read and agreed to the published version of the manuscript.

Funding: This work was partly supported by the Japan Agency for Medical Research and Development (AMED) under grant number JP19ek0109278 (Chief Investigator: Yoichi Matsubara), and grant numbers JP19gk0110040, and JP21gk0110050 (Chief Investigator: Go Tajima).

Institutional Review Board Statement: The study was conducted according to the guidelines of the Declaration of Helsinki, and approved by the ethics committee of Hiroshima University (E-1522, 8 February 2019).

Informed Consent Statement: Informed consent was obtained from the parents of all subjects involved in the study.

Data Availability Statement: The data that support the findings of this study are available from the corresponding author, Go Tajima.

Acknowledgments: The authors would like to thank Osamu Sakamoto for performing MTHFR genetic analysis. We thank Sarah Williams from Edanz Group (https://jp.edanz.com/ac, accessed on 1 July 2021) for editing a draft of this manuscript.

Conflicts of Interest: The authors declare no conflict of interest.

References

1. Huemer, M.; Diodato, D.; Schwahn, B.; Schiff, M.; Bandeira, A.; Benoist, J.F.; Burlina, A.; Cerone, R.; Couce, M.L.; Cazorla, A.G.; et al. Guidelines for diagnosis and management of the cobalamin-related remethylation disorders cblC, cblD, cblE, cblF, cblG, cblJ and MTHFR deficiency. *J. Inherit. Metab. Dis.* **2017**, *40*, 21–48. [CrossRef] [PubMed]
2. Keller, R.; Chrastina, P.; Pavlíková, M.; Gouveia, S.; Ribes, A.; Kölker, S.; Blom, H.J.; Baumgartner, M.R.; Bártl, J.; Dionisi-Vici, C.; et al. Newborn screening for homocystinurias: Recent recommendations versus current practice. *J. Inherit. Metab. Dis.* **2019**, *42*, 128–139. [CrossRef] [PubMed]
3. Huemer, M.; Kozich, V.; Rinaldo, P.; Baumgartner, M.R.; Merinero, B.; Pasquini, E.; Ribes, A.; Blom, H.J. Newborn screening for homocystinurias and methylation disorders: Systematic review and proposed guidelines. *J. Inherit. Metab. Dis.* **2015**, *38*, 1007–1019. [CrossRef]

4. Diekman, E.F.; Koning, T.J.; Verhoeven-Duif, N.M.; Rovers, M.M.; Hasselt, P.M. Survival and psychomotor development with early betaine treatment in patients with severe methylenetetrahydrofolate reductase deficiency. *JAMA Neurol.* **2014**, *71*, 188–194. [CrossRef] [PubMed]
5. Ito, Y.; Sakakibara, T.; Nishiku, T. Early treatment using betaine and methionine for a neonate with MTHFR deficiency. *Pediatrics Int.* **2019**, *61*, 1265–1266. [CrossRef]
6. Adams, J.D.; Bender, H.A.; Miley-Åkerstedt, A.; Frempong, T.; Schrager, N.L.; Patel, K.; Naidich, T.P.; Stein, V.; Spat, J.; Towns, S.; et al. Neurologic and neurodevelopmental phenotypes in young children with early-treated combined methylmalonic acidemia and homocystinuria, cobalamin C type. *Mol. Genet. Metab.* **2014**, *110*, 241–247. [CrossRef] [PubMed]
7. Wong, D.; Tortorelli, S.; Bishop, L.; Sellars, E.A.; Schimmenti, L.A.; Gallant, N.; Prada, C.E.; Hopkin, R.J.; Leslie, N.D.; Berry, S.A.; et al. Outcomes of four patients with homocysteine remethylation disorders detected by newborn screening. *Genet. Med.* **2016**, *18*, 162–167. [CrossRef] [PubMed]
8. Ono, H.; Tajima, G.; Shigematsu, Y.; Hata, I.; Hara, K.; Sakura, N.; Yoshii. A case of vitamin B_{12} responsive methylmalonic acidemia who developed clinical manifestation following norovirus infection with negative results in newborn mass screening with tandem mass spectrometry. *Jpn. J. Neonatal Screen.* **2014**, *24*, 49–56. (In Japanese)
9. Kagawa, R.; Tajima, G.; Maeda, T.; Hara, K.; Nishimura, Y.; Yoshii, C.; Shigematsu, Y. Preliminary study on newborn screening for inborn errors of cobalamin metabolism by hypomethioninemia. *Jpn. J. Neonatal Screen.* **2019**, *29*, 51–56. (In Japanese)
10. Gavrilov, D.K.; Piazza, A.L.; Pino, G.; Turgeon, C.; Matern, D.; Oglesbee, D.; Raymond, K.; Tortorelli, S.; Rinaldo, P. The combined impact of CLIR post-analytical tools and second tier testing on the performance of newborn screening for disorders of propionate, methionine, and cobalamin metabolism. *Int. J. Neonatal Screen.* **2020**, *6*, 33. [CrossRef]
11. Shigematsu, Y.; Hata, I.; Kikawa, Y.; Mayumia, M.; Tanaka, Y.; Sudo, M.; Kado, N. Modifications in electrospray tandem mass spectrometry for a neonatal-screening pilot study in Japan. *J. Chromatogr. B Biomed. Sci. Appl.* **1999**, *731*, 97–103. [CrossRef]
12. Rozmaric, T.; Mitulovic, G.; Konstantopoulou, V.; Goeschl, B.; Huemer, M.; Plecko, B.; Spenger, J.; Wortmann, S.B.; Scholl-Bürgi, S.; Karall, D.; et al. Elevated homocysteine after elevated propionylcarnitine or low methionine in newborn screening is highly predictive for low vitamin B12 and holo-transcobalamin levels in newborns. *Diagnostics* **2020**, *10*, 626. [CrossRef] [PubMed]
13. Gramer, M.; Hoffmann, J.F.; Feyh, P.; Monostori, P.; Mütze, U.; Posset, R.; Weiss, K.H.; Hoffmann, G.F.; Okun, J.G. Newborn screening for vitamin B12 deficiency in Germany—Strategies, results, and Public Health Implications. *J. Pediatrics* **2020**, *216*, 165–172. [CrossRef] [PubMed]
14. HAbu-El-Haija, A.; Mendelsohn, B.A.; Duncan, J.L.; Moore, A.T.; Glenn, O.A.; Weisiger, K.; Gallagher, R.C. Cobalamin D deficiency identified through newborn screening. In *JIMD Reports*; Springer: Berlin/Heidelberg, Germany, 2019; Volume 44, pp. 73–77. [CrossRef]
15. Hannibal, L.; Lysne, V.; Bjørke-Monsen, A.L.; Behringer, S.; Grünert, S.C.; Spiekerkoetter, U.; Jacobsen, D.W.; Blom, H.J. Biomarkers and algorithms for the diagnosis of vitamin B12 deficiency. *Front. Mol. Biosci.* **2016**, *3*, 27. [CrossRef] [PubMed]
16. Tortorelli, S.; Turgeon, C.T.; Lim, J.S.; Baumgart, S.; Day-Salvatore, D.L.; Abdenur, J.; Bernstein, J.A.; Lorey, F.; Lichter-Konecki, U.; Oglesbee, D.; et al. Two-tier approach to the newborn screening of methylenetetrahydrofolate reductase deficiency and other remethylation disorders with tandem mass spectrometry. *J. Pediatrics* **2010**, *157*, 271–275. [CrossRef] [PubMed]
17. Shigematsu, Y.; Hata, I.; Tajima, G. Useful second-tier tests in expanded newborn screening of isovaleric acidemia and methylmalonic aciduria. *J. Inherit. Metab. Dis.* **2010**, *33*, S283–S288. [CrossRef] [PubMed]

Article

Spinal Muscular Atrophy: Diagnosis, Incidence, and Newborn Screening in Japan

Tomokazu Kimizu [1], Shinobu Ida [2], Kentaro Okamoto [3], Hiroyuki Awano [4], Emma Tabe Eko Niba [5], Yogik Onky Silvana Wijaya [5], Shin Okazaki [6], Hideki Shimomura [7], Tomoko Lee [7], Koji Tominaga [8], Shin Nabatame [8], Toshio Saito [9], Takashi Hamazaki [10], Norio Sakai [11], Kayoko Saito [12], Haruo Shintaku [10], Kandai Nozu [4], Yasuhiro Takeshima [7], Kazumoto Iijima [4,13], Hisahide Nishio [5,14,]* and Masakazu Shinohara [5]

1. Department of Pediatric Neurology, Osaka Women's and Children's Hospital, 840 Murodocho, Izumi 594-1101, Japan; kimizu@wch.opho.jp
2. Department of Laboratory Medicine, Osaka Women's and Children's Hospital, 840 Murodocho, Izumi 594-1101, Japan; idas@wch.opho.jp
3. Department of Pediatrics, Ehime Prefectural Imabari Hospital, 4-5-5 Ishiicho, Imabari 794-0006, Japan; kentaro206@gmail.com
4. Department of Pediatrics, Kobe University Graduate School of Medicine, 7-5-1 Kusunoki-cho, Kobe 650-0017, Japan; awahiro@med.kobe-u.ac.jp (H.A.); nozu@med.kobe-u.ac.jp (K.N.); iijima@med.kobe-u.ac.jp (K.I.)
5. Department of Community Medicine and Social Healthcare Science, Kobe University Graduate School of Medicine, 7-5-1 Kusunoki-cho, Kobe 650-0017, Japan; niba@med.kobe-u.ac.jp (E.T.E.N.); yogik.onky@gmail.com (Y.O.S.W.); mashino@med.kobe-u.ac.jp (M.S.)
6. Department of Pediatric Neurology, Children's Medical Center, Osaka City General Hospital, 2-13-22 Miyakojimahondori, Osaka 534-0021, Japan; sokazaki2009@gmail.com
7. Department of Pediatrics, Hyogo College of Medicine, 1-1 Mukogawacho, Nishinomiya 663-8501, Japan; shimomura.ped@gmail.com (H.S.); leeleetomo@me.com (T.L.); ytake@hyo-med.ac.jp (Y.T.)
8. Department of Pediatrics, Osaka University Graduate School of Medicine, 2-2 Yamadaoka, Suita 565-0871, Japan; yasuhito@ped.med.osaka-u.ac.jp (K.T.); nabatames@ped.med.osaka-u.ac.jp (S.N.)
9. Division of Child Neurology, Department of Neurology, National Hospital Organization Osaka Toneyama Medical Center, 5-1-1 Toneyama, Toyonaka 560-8552, Japan; saito.toshio.cq@mail.hosp.go.jp
10. Department of Pediatrics, Osaka City University Graduate School of Medicine, 1-4-3 Asahi-machi, Osaka 545-8585, Japan; hammer@med.osaka-cu.ac.jp (T.H.); shintakuh@med.osaka-cu.ac.jp (H.S.)
11. Child Healthcare and Genetic Science Laboratory, Division of Health Sciences, Osaka University Graduate School of Medicine, 2-2 Yamadaoka, Suita 565-0871, Japan; norio@ped.med.osaka-u.ac.jp
12. Institute of Medical Genetics, Tokyo Women's Medical University, 8-1 Kawadacho, Tokyo 162-0054, Japan; saito.kayoko@twmu.ac.jp
13. Hyogo Prefectural Kobe Children's Hospital, 1-6-7 Minatojima Minamimachi, Kobe 650-0047, Japan
14. Faculty of Medical Rehabilitation, Kobe Gakuin University, 518 Arise Ikawadani-cho, Kobe 651-2180, Japan
* Correspondence: nishio@reha.kobegakuin.ac.jp; Tel.: +81-789-745-073

Abstract: Spinal muscular atrophy (SMA) is a genetic neuromuscular disorder that causes degeneration of anterior horn cells in the human spinal cord and subsequent loss of motor neurons. The severe form of SMA is among the genetic diseases with the highest infant mortality. Although SMA has been considered incurable, newly developed drugs—nusinersen and onasemnogene abeparvovec—improve the life prognoses and motor functions of affected infants. To maximize the efficacy of these drugs, treatments should be started at the pre-symptomatic stage of SMA. Thus, newborn screening for SMA is now strongly recommended. Herein, we provide some data based on our experience of SMA diagnosis by genetic testing in Japan. A total of 515 patients suspected of having SMA or another lower motor neuron disease were tested. Among these patients, 228 were diagnosed as having SMA with survival motor neuron 1 (*SMN1*) deletion. We analyzed the distribution of clinical subtypes and ages at genetic testing in the *SMN1*-deleted patients, and estimated the SMA incidence based on data from Osaka and Hyogo prefectures, Japan. Our data showed that confirmed diagnosis by genetic testing was notably delayed, and the estimated incidence was 1 in 30,000–40,000 live births, which seemed notably lower than in other countries. These findings suggest that many diagnosis-delayed or undiagnosed cases may be present in Japan. To prevent this, newborn screening programs for SMA (SMA-NBS) need to be implemented in all Japanese prefectures. In this article, we also introduce our pilot study for SMA-NBS in Osaka Prefecture.

Keywords: spinal muscular atrophy; *SMN1*; deletion; incidence; newborn screening

1. Introduction

Spinal muscular atrophy (SMA) is a genetic neuromuscular disorder that causes degeneration of anterior horn cells in the human spinal cord and subsequent loss of motor neurons [1]. According to a previous report, it has a prevalence of approximately 1–2 per 100,000 individuals and an incidence of around 1 in 10,000 live births [2]. Two SMA-related genes mapped to chromosome 5q13, survival motor neuron 1 (*SMN1*) and survival motor neuron 2 (*SMN2*) [3], which are highly homologous, were reported in 1995. *SMN1* is now considered as a gene causative of SMA. More than 90% of SMA patients are homozygous for *SMN1* deletion, while the rest are compound heterozygous for a deleted *SMN1* allele and a mutated *SMN1* allele [3]. In contrast, *SMN2* is considered to be a modifying factor of the SMA phenotype because a higher copy number of *SMN2* may be related to a milder SMA phenotype [4].

SMA is clinically divided into five subtypes [5]: Type 0 (the most severe form with onset in the prenatal period; severe respiratory problems after birth, and, typically, death within weeks of birth), Type I (Werdnig–Hoffmann disease; a severe form with onset before 6 months of age; the inability to sit unsupported), Type II (Dubowitz disease; an intermediate form with onset before 18 months of age; the ability to sit unaided but not to stand or walk), Type III (Kugelberg–Welander disease; a mild form with onset after 18 months of age; the ability to stand and walk unaided), and Type IV (the mildest form with onset after 30 years of age). SMA type I is a genetic disease with high infant mortality [6]. Many patients with SMA type I die of respiratory insufficiency by 2 years of age, when respiratory support is not available [7]. Meanwhile, patients with types II, III and IV are also forced to lead lives with limited motor function, showing various levels of severity.

Until recently, SMA was considered to be incurable. However, treatments for this disease are emerging. In 2016, the United States Food and Drug Administration (FDA) approved nusinersen (Spinraza®, Biogen, Cambridge, MA), the first drug designated to treat SMA. Nusinersen is an *SMN2*-directed antisense oligonucleotide drug, which alters *SMN2*'s pre-mRNA splicing pattern to produce more SMN protein in the motor neuron cells in SMA [8]. In 2019, the FDA approved onasemnogene abeparvovec (Zolgensma®, AveXis Inc, Bannockburn, IL) as the second drug for treating SMA. Onasemnogene abeparvovec is an adeno-associated viral vector-based gene therapy designed to deliver a functional copy of the human *SMN* gene to the motor neuron cells of SMA patients [9]. The Japanese Ministry of Health, Labour and Welfare approved nusinersen in 2017 and approved onasemnogene abeparvovec in 2020. These new drugs improve the life prognoses and motor functions of infants affected by SMA.

According to early reports of clinical trials, nusinersen and onasemnogene abeparvovec helped patients to reach milestones in their motor function development and increased their likelihood of survival [10,11]. The most recent report of the clinical trials with these drugs showed that early treatment, especially at the pre-symptomatic stage, resulted in better outcomes in SMA patients; even SMA type I patients became able to stand and walk [12,13].

Delayed diagnosis leads to delayed treatment, resulting in limited effects on the clinical phenotype [10,11]. Thus, newborn screening (NBS) for SMA is now strongly recommended. As more than 90% of SMA patients are homozygous for *SMN1* deletion, as mentioned above, the presence or absence of *SMN1* can be a good marker for SMA screening. In Japan, NBS programs for SMA have just started in some areas, including Osaka, Hyogo, Chiba, Aichi, and Kumamoto prefectures. However, at present, the number of infants tested in the screening programs is insufficient to obtain an estimate of the incidence of SMA in Japan.

According to a global overview of the current situation of NBS for SMA (SMA-NBS) [14], nine SMA-NBS programs performed in various countries have so far detected 288 newborns with SMA out of 3,674,277 newborns screened. The annual proportion of newborns to be screened for SMA in the coming years is expected to increase steadily [14]. Our SMA-NBS programs will cover all newborns throughout Japan in the near future.

In this article, we first report our experience of genetic diagnosis based on testing for *SMN1* deletion. Second, we present the estimated incidence of SMA based on data from Osaka and Hyogo prefectures, Japan. Third, we describe a pilot study for SMA-NBS in Osaka Prefecture and discuss the need to implement SMA-NBS programs throughout Japan.

2. Patients and Methods

2.1. Diagnosis of SMA

A total of 515 patients from 36 out of 47 prefectures in Japan were referred to the Department of Community Medicine and Social Healthcare Science, Kobe University Graduate School of Medicine, in the period from 1996 to 2019. These patients were suspected of having SMA or another lower motor neuron disease (LMND). Their ages varied from several days after birth to 63 years. Infants, toddlers, and children presented with such indications as delayed developmental milestones, respiratory problems, and muscle weakness. Meanwhile, adult patients showed symptoms including walking disability and muscle weakness.

Prior to genetic analysis, written informed consent was obtained from the patients or their parents/guardians. All procedures were reviewed and approved by the Ethics Committee of Kobe University Graduate School of Medicine, and were performed in accordance with the ethical standards laid down in the Declaration of Helsinki.

Genetic testing was performed according to PCR-enzyme digestion [15] and/or multiplex ligation-dependent probe amplification analysis (MLPA) methods [16]. Copy numbers of *SMN1* and *SMN2* were determined in accordance with the methods of Harada et al. [17] and Tran et al. [18], and the MLPA method.

2.2. Implementation of SMA-NBS

In Osaka Prefecture, a pilot study for SMA-NBS was initiated in February 2021. This pilot study was approved by the Institutional Review Board of Osaka Women's and Children's Hospital. After obtaining written informed consent from the parents, DBS samples were collected from their offspring within 4–6 days after birth at the maternity hospital. Then, they were sent to Osaka Women's and Children's Hospital, and SMA-NBS was performed there using $5'$–$3'$ exonuclease-based real-time PCR with fluorescent probes [19].

2.3. Statistical Analysis

To compare the *SMN2* copy numbers among SMA subtypes, Welch's *t*-test was used, and to compare the proportions of confirmed diagnosis at the proper timing between SMA type I and type II, the chi-squared test was used. For these analyses, we used Microsoft Excel with the add-in software Statcel 4 (The Publisher OMS Ltd., Tokyo, Japan). A *p*-value less than 0.05 was considered to indicate statistical significance.

The incidence of SMA was defined as the number of newborn infants with the disease in a year in the population, and was expressed as the number of affected infants per 100,000 live births. The 95% confidence intervals of the incidence were calculated based on the Poisson distribution using Microsoft Excel. Population data were provided by the Statistics Bureau, Ministry of Internal Affairs and Communications of Japan.

3. Results

3.1. Genetic Analysis of Patients Suspected of Having SMA

3.1.1. *SMN1* Deletion Test

Among 515 patients who were referred to our laboratory in the period from 1996 to 2019, we confirmed 228 cases as having SMA with homozygous *SMN1* deletion [15]. The remaining 287 cases retained at least one *SMN1* copy. Subsequently, 33 out of the 287 patients with SMA- or LMND-like symptoms were shown to carry only one *SMN1* copy, while 13 out of these 33 carried a deleterious *SMN1* mutation causing SMA. Our data demonstrated 44.3% of the 515 patients (228/515) carried a homozygous *SMN1* deletion, 2.5% (13/515) carried an intragenic mutation (or a subtle mutation) and an *SMN1* deletion, whereas 53.2% (274/515) remained undiagnosed at the genetic level. Thus, *SMN1*-related SMA may account for half of the patients with SMA-like or LMND-like symptoms. To clarify the causative gene abnormalities in the patients with non-*SMN1*-related SMA, targeted resequencing analysis using next-generation sequencing technology may be essential [20,21].

3.1.2. Distribution of SMA Subtype and *SMN2* Copy Number

We determined the subtype distribution in the patients tested in our laboratory. Here, we used the data of 221 SMA patients with homozygous *SMN1* deletion for whom clinical information was available. Among these 221 patients tested in our laboratory, 42.1% (93/221) were diagnosed with SMA type I, 32.1% (71/221) with type II, 20.8% (46/221) with type III, and 5.0% (11/221) with type IV. Three families with affected siblings were included in our database. Each family had two affected siblings with subtype concordance (type II or type III).

Next, we determined the *SMN2* copy number in 204 out of 221 SMA patients with homozygous *SMN1* deletion (83 out of 93 patients with SMA type I, 70 out of 71 patients with SMA type II, 40 out of 46 patients with SMA type III, and 11 out of 11 patients with SMA type IV). A high *SMN2* copy number modifies the phenotype of SMA patients with homozygous deletion of *SMN1* [5]. Our database of SMA patients with homozygous *SMN1* deletion supported the conventional observation of a low *SMN2* copy number resulting in a severe phenotype and a high copy number potentially being related to a milder one (Table 1). Patients with SMA type I usually carry only two copies of *SMN2*, while SMA type II is usually associated with three copies. SMA type III patients have three to four copies, and SMA type IV patients usually have four or more copies. A high *SMN2* copy number may improve the survival outcomes and motor function.

Table 1. SMA types and copy number of *SMN2* in *SMN1*-deleted patients.

Copy Number	1	2	3	4	Mean ± SD
Type I (n = 83)	1	66	16	0	2.18 ± 0.64
Type II (n = 70)	0	3	67	0	2.96 ± 0.09
Type III (n = 40)	0	2	25	13	3.28 ± 0.15
Type IV (n = 11)	0	0	1	10	3.91 ± 0.58
Total (n = 204)	1	71	109	23	

Welch's *t*-test was used to determine differences between groups. All of the differences between groups were significant with $p < 0.01$.

3.2. Age of Genetic Testing among SMA Patients

Since *SMN1* was identified as an SMA-causing gene in 1995, genetic testing, especially testing for the *SMN1* deletion, has been widely used to confirm the diagnosis of SMA [5]. The age at genetic testing of the patients referred to our laboratory is shown in Table 2. In this analysis, we used the data of 142 SMA patients with homozygous *SMN1* deletion (84 type I, 43 type II, and 15 type III). The remaining SMA patients were excluded because the onset age information was missing. These patients were born between January 1996 and September 2018. The mean ages at genetic testing were 11.0 months old (standard deviation (SD) ± 23.7) for type I, 77.3 months old (SD ± 79.9) for type II, and 85.1 months old (SD ± 79.1) for type III.

Table 2. Age and timing of confirmed diagnosis by genetic testing.

	(A) Age at Genetic Testing (Months)		
	Mean Age (SD)	Median (Range)	Interquartile Range
Type I (n = 84)	11.0 (23.7)	5 (0 to 182)	7
Type II (n = 43)	77.3 (79.9)	29 (13 to 262)	122
Type III (n = 15)	85.1 (79.1)	45 (22 to 239)	79
	(B) Timing at Genetic Diagnosis (Months)		
	Proper Timing	Slightly Delayed Timing	Notably Delayed Timing
Type I (n = 84)	<6 m	6 to 12 m	>12 m
	55 (65.5%)	15 (17.9%)	14 (16.7%)
Type II (n = 43)	<18 m	18 to 30 m	>30 m
	9 (20.9%)	13 (30.2%)	21 (48.8%)

The exact ages of onset of many patients were not available in this study. Thus, we could not determine the exact duration between onset and genetic testing. Instead, we calculated the proportions of cases with a "proper," "slightly delayed," or "notably delayed" timing of genetic testing for the confirmed diagnosis of SMA type I and type II, as shown in Table 2. As for SMA type III, we excluded it from the "timing of genetic testing" analysis because it is a late-onset and slowly progressive disease.

The definitions of "proper", "slightly delayed," and "notably delayed" timing were as follows: (1) for SMA type I, "proper" timing of diagnosis is within 6 months after birth, "slightly delayed" timing is between 6 and 12 months, and "notably delayed" timing is more than 12 months; (2) for SMA type II, "proper" timing of diagnosis is earlier than 18 months, "slightly delayed" timing is between 18 and 24 months, and "notably delayed" timing is more than 24 months.

Overall, confirmed diagnosis of SMA was slightly delayed or notably delayed in 63 out of 127 (50.0%) patients (29 out of 84 type I patients, and 34 out of 43 type II patients). Only 20.9% of type II patients were diagnosed at the proper timing, which was a markedly lower rate than that of type I patients (65.5%). There was a significant difference in the number of confirmed diagnoses at the proper timing between type I and type II patients ($p < 0.01$).

3.3. Epidemiological Analysis of SMA in Osaka and Hyogo Prefectures

We estimated the incidence of SMA using the number of SMA-affected infants who were born or SMA-affected fetuses who were aborted in Osaka and Hyogo prefectures from 2007 to 2016 and diagnosed as having SMA by genetic testing within this period (Table 3).

Table 3. Incidence of SMA in Osaka and Hyogo Prefectures.

Live Birth (n = 1,197,156)	Affected Individuals		
	Infants	Fetuses	Total
No. of types I, II and III	28	9	37
Incidence *	2.34 (95%CI: −0.66, 4.53)		3.09 (95%CI: −0.36, 5.20)
No. of type I	14	7	21
Incidence *	1.08 (95%CI: −0.95, 3.20)		1.32 (95%CI: −0.84, 3.92)

* Incidence in 100,000 of population (study period, 2007 to 2016).

The number of newborn infants with SMA (including types I, II, and III) was 28 out of 1,197,156 live births. We thus estimated that the incidence of SMA was 2.34 per 100,000 live births (95% CI: −0.66, 4.53)—that is, ~1 in 40,000. We also had information on aborted fetuses with a prenatal diagnosis of SMA. When this number was added to the number of newborns with SMA, the estimated incidence of SMA was 3.09 per 100,000 live births (95% CI: −0.36, 5.20)—that is, ~1 in 30,000.

The number of newborn infants with SMA type I was 14 out of 1,197,156 live births. We thus calculated that the estimated incidence of SMA type I was 1.08 per 100,000 live births (95% CI: −0.95, 3.20)—that is, ~1 in 100,000. When the number of aborted infants with a prenatal diagnosis of SMA type I was added to the number of newborn infants with SMA, the estimated incidence of SMA type I was 1.32 per 100,000 live births (95% CI: −0.84, 3.92)—that is, ~1 in 80,000. Here, the diagnosis of SMA type I in the aborted fetuses was based on the clinical subtype of the patients in the same family. We analyzed all cases of SMA-affected fetuses and their affected sibling in our laboratory.

3.4. Implementation of SMA-NBS in Osaka Prefecture

More than 10,000 new DBS samples from neonates born in Osaka Prefecture were tested in the pilot study for an SMA-NBS program as of 17 May 2021. The assay tested for the presence/absence of *SMN1*. All DBS samples tested negative for SMA.

4. Discussion

4.1. SMA Subtype and SMN2 Copy Number in Japanese SMA Patients

Almost all data reported from groups around the world, including ours, show similar tendencies (Table 4). Specifically, type I patients predominate (40%–60% of all SMA patients), while type IV patients are very rare (less than 5% of all SMA patients) in all populations. Roughly speaking, half of SMA patients are type I, while the other half are types II and III.

A high *SMN2* copy number modifies the phenotype of SMA patients with homozygous deletion of *SMN1* [5]. Our database of SMA patients with homozygous *SMN1* deletion supported the conventional observation that a low *SMN2* copy number results in a severe phenotype and a high copy number may be related to milder SMA phenotypes (Table 1). However, we did not observe such a tendency in all SMA patients with an intragenic *SMN1* mutation in our previous studies [22,23].

Among the SMA patients with an intragenic mutation, some with a milder phenotype carried only a single *SMN2* copy, while others with a severe phenotype carried three *SMN2* copies. For patients with an intragenic *SMN1* mutation, we cannot conclude that clinical severity is inversely correlated with the *SMN2* copy number. The locations and types of intragenic *SMN1* mutations may make more significant contributions to the clinical phenotype than the *SMN2* copy number.

Table 4. Subtype distribution in countries.

Country	Total Patient Number	Type I	Type II	Type III	Type IV	Unknown
Germany (1999) [24]	525 (a)	270 (51.4%)	124 (23.6%)	131 (25.0%)	*	*
Saudi Arabia (2003) [25]	121 (a)	60 (49.6%)	26 (21.5%)	35 (28.9%)	*	*
South Africa (2007) [26]	24 (a) (White)	15 (62.5%)	4 (type II & III) (16.6%)		*	5 (20.9%)
	92 (a) (Black)	48 (52.2%)	39 (types II & III) (42.4%)		*	5 (5.4%)

Table 4. Cont.

Country	Total Patient Number	Type I	Type II	Type III	Type IV	Unknown
Malaysia (2007) [27]	24 (a)	10 (41.7%)	11 (45.8%)	3 (12.5%)	*	*
Vietnam (2008) [18]	34 (a)	13 (38.2%)	11 (32.4%)	10 (29.4%)	*	*
Spain (2018) [4]	625 (a)	272 (43.5%)	186 (29.7%)	167 (26.7%)	*	*
Cure SMA (2018) [28]	1966 (b) (Worldwide)	1021 (51.9%)	635 (32.3%)	310 (15.8%)	*	*
Japan (2019) [29]	486 (a)	164 (33.7%)	210 (43.2%)	99 (20.4%)	7 (1.4%)	6 (1.0%)
China (2020) [30]	419 (a)	177 (45.6%)	126 (27.4%)	100 (23.2%)	16 (3.8%)	*
Greece (2020) [31]	361 (a)	156 (43.2%)	93 (25.8%)	107 (29.6%)	5 (1.4%)	*
Japan (This study)	221 (a)	93 (42.1%)	71 (32.1%)	46 (20.8%)	11 (5.0%)	*

(a) Patients confirmed diagnosis by genetic testing. (b) Self-identified patients registered in the Cure SMA database, one of the largest patient-reported data repositories on SMA patients worldwide. About 59.0% of affected individuals in the U.S.A. are registered in the Cure SMA database. * There is no description in the original article.

4.2. Age at Genetic Testing among Japanese SMA Patients

Upon comparison with the findings in previous reports from other countries, we conclude that SMA diagnosis may still be delayed in Japan. According to a review of 21 studies reported in the literature by Lin et al. [32] in 2015, the weighted mean ages of genetic diagnosis were 6.3 months old (SD ± 2.2), 20.7 months old (SD ± 2.6), and 50.3 months old (SD ± 12.9), for types I, II, and III, respectively. Pera et al. also reported a study on the age of genetic diagnosis of SMA in Italy [33]. The cohort included 480 patients (191 type I, 210 type II, and 79 type III). The mean ages of genetic diagnosis were 4.70 months old (SD ± 2.82) for type I, 15.6 months old (SD ± 5.88) for type II, and 4.34 years old (SD ± 4.01) for type III.

In our study in Japan, a confirmed diagnosis of SMA type II was often delayed. Only 20.9% of type II patients were diagnosed at the proper timing, while 65.5% of type I patients were diagnosed at the proper timing. This may reflect the respiratory-stable condition of infants or toddlers with type II SMA, which does not require an urgent diagnosis. Specifically, SMA type II infants are usually respiratory-stable and do not need respiratory support. In contrast, infants with type I SMA often suffer from respiratory insufficiency.

4.3. Incidence of SMA in Hyogo and Osaka Prefectures

Few studies on the incidence of SMA in Japan have been performed. According to a survey by Imaizumi based on death certificate records [34], the incidence of SMA type I between 1979 and 1996 was estimated to be 1.2 per 100,000 live births in Japan. This report used only clinically diagnosed cases, and some cases with SMA type I were not included because other disease names were likely used on the death certificate.

According to a report based on a survey by Okamoto et al. [29], the incidence of infantile SMA (type I) was estimated to be 2.70 per 100,000 live births (95% CI: 0.1–5.4) on Shikoku Island, Japan, between 2011 and 2015.

We also estimated the incidence of SMA using the number of SMA-affected infants who were born or SMA-affected fetuses who were aborted in Hyogo and Osaka prefectures from 2007 to 2016 (Table 3). Based on our data in this study, the incidences of SMA (total) and SMA type I were estimated to be 3.09 per 100,000 live births (95% CI: −0.36, 5.20) and 1.32 per 100,000 live births (95% CI: −0.84, 3.92), respectively.

The incidence of SMA among Asian populations is lower than that in Western countries. Belter et al., who analyzed the Cure SMA membership database, described in their report [28] that, "Hispanics and Asians have a lower projected SMA incidence than the general population, and it follows that states with a higher proportion of Hispanics and Asians would have a lower overall incidence of SMA than the general population."

Even so, our estimate of the incidence of SMA in Japan was notably lower than the data reported from another Asian country, Taiwan [39] (Table 5). We are thus concerned that many SMA patients may be overlooked or misdiagnosed in Japan.

Table 5. Incidence of SMA in various countries.

(A) Incidences of SMA Based on Survey Research					
SMA Types I, II & III					
Country	Study Period	Cases Detected	Live Births	Incidence (In 100,000)	Reference
Sweden	1980–2006	45	531,746	8.5 (a)	(2009) [35]
Poland	1998–2005	304	2,963,783	10.3	(2010) [36]
Europe	2011–2015	3776	22,325,221	11.9 (b)	(2017) [2]
Japan (c)	2007–2016	37(d)	1,197,178	3.1	This study
SMA Type I					
Country	Study Period	Cases Detected	Live Births	Incidence (In 100,000)	Reference
Sweden	1980–2006	19	531,746	3.6	(2009) [35]
Estonia	1994–2003	9	129,832	6.9	(2006) [37]
Poland	1998–2005	209	2,963,783	7.1	(2010) [36]
Japan (e)	2011–2015	4	147,950	2.7	(2019) [29]
Japan (c)	2007–2016	21(d)	1,197,178	1.3	This study
(B) Incidences of SMA Based on Newborn Screening Programs					
SMA Types I, II & III					
Country	Study Period	Cases	Live Births	Incidence (In 100,000)	Reference
U.S. (Ohio)	–2009	4	40,103	10.0	(2010) [38]
Taiwan	2014–2016	7	120,267	5.8	(2017) [39]
U.S. (New York City)	2016–2017	1	3826	26.1 (f)	(2018) [40]
Japan	2018–2019	0	4157	0.0 (f)	(2019) [41]
Germany	2018–2020	43	297,163	14.5	(2021) [42]
Australia	2018–2020	18	202,388	8.9	(2021) [43]
U.S. (North Carolina)	2018–2020	1	12,065	8.3	(2021) [44]

(a) All patients were younger than 16 years old. (b) Median incidence of several countries in Europe. (c) Hyogo and Osaka Prefectures in Japan. (d) Case number included affected infants and fetuses. (e) Ehime, Kagawa, Tokushima and Kochi Prefectures in Japan (f) The number of newborns tested in the SMA-NBS program was too small to obtain precise incidence of SMA patients.

4.4. Initiation of NBS for SMA in Japan

In Japan, a mandatory NBS program for inherited disorders is conducted using DBS samples from infants. All municipalities have mandatory with defined opt-out policies for parents. At the initiation of nationwide implementation of this program in 1977, only five diseases (phenylketonuria, galactosemia, maple syrup urine, homocystinuria, and histidinemia) were screened.

Since tandem mass spectrometry analysis was introduced into the NBS program as a first-line screening methodology in the early 2000s, many inborn errors of metabolism have been added to the list of target diseases for primary screening. Twenty diseases are now included among the screening targets.

Recently, many families of patients suffering from inherited disorders such as SMA, severe combined immunodeficiency disease (SCID) and lysosomal storage disease have demanded for the inclusion of such diseases in the NBS program. At the time of writing this, such expanded screening programs are about to start as optional programs in prefectures including Osaka, Hyogo, Chiba, Aichi, and Kumamoto.

We have also been engaged in developing new SMA screening technologies using DBS since 2010 [41,45–47]. The most sophisticated technology that we have developed to date is an allele-specific real-time PCR with short primers (10–12 mers), which we named "modified competitive oligonucleotide priming (mCOP)-PCR" [41,47]. We applied this mCOP-PCR technology to a prospective SMA screening study using DBS samples from 4157 Japanese newborns [41]. All DBS samples tested were negative, but there were no screening failures or false positives [41]. These results indicated that our system is applicable to SMA-NBS programs in any region or country. Nonetheless, we still think that our system should be investigated and reported on further because we are aiming for implementation in all prefectures in Japan and other countries.

Note: during the submission of this manuscript, it was reported that an infant with SMA had been detected by a pilot study for the NBS program in Kumamoto Prefecture [48]. The infant was reported to be treated with onasemnogene abeparvovec.

5. Conclusions

In this paper, we have described our experience of SMA diagnosis and the estimated the incidence of SMA based on data from Osaka and Hyogo prefectures, Japan. Upon comparing our data to findings previously reported from other countries, the diagnosis of SMA as confirmed by genetic testing was delayed in many Japanese patients. In addition, the estimated incidence of SMA was notably lower than that reported in other countries. These results suggested that many SMA patients in Japan may be overlooked or misdiagnosed. SMA-NBS would allow SMA patients to undergo early treatment with the potential for the maximal therapeutic benefit. Thus, there is an urgent need to implement a diagnostic system incorporating SMA-NBS in Japan. In addition, if an SMA screening system such as SMA-NBS becomes available to current Japanese patients with SMA-like or LMND-like symptoms, a large proportion of such patients may be diagnosed as having SMA and could access the new therapies. Finally, we hope that SMA-NBS programs will soon be implemented in all prefectures in Japan.

Author Contributions: Conceptualization, H.N. and M.S.; methodology, H.N.; formal analysis, H.N., E.T.E.N. and Y.O.S.W.; investigation, H.A., S.O., H.S. (Hideki Shimomura), T.L., K.T. and S.N.; resources, H.A., S.O., H.S. (Hideki Shimomura), T.L., K.T. and S.N.; data curation, H.N., E.T.E.N. and Y.O.S.W.; writing—original draft preparation, T.K., K.O. and H.N.; writing—review and editing, H.N., T.S. and Y.T.; supervision, H.N. and K.S.; project administration, S.I., T.H., H.S. (Haruo Shintaku), N.S., Y.T., K.N. and K.I.; funding acquisition, H.N. All authors have read and agreed to the published version of the manuscript.

Funding: This research was supported by the Ministry of Education, Culture, Sports, Science and Technology, Japan, Grant No. 20K08197.

Institutional Review Board Statement: This study was conducted in accordance with the Declaration of Helsinki, and approved by the Ethics Committee of Kobe University Graduate School of Medicine (protocol code: 1089, 5 October 2018) and the Institutional Review Board of Osaka Women's and Children's Hospital (protocol code: 1361, 1 September 2020).

Informed Consent Statement: Informed consent was obtained from all subjects involved in the study.

Data Availability Statement: The data presented in this paper are available on request from the corresponding author. Publicly available datasets were also analyzed in this study.

Acknowledgments: We are indebted to all SMA-affected patients and their parents/guardians who participated in this study. We are grateful to Seiji Yamaguchi for his helpful comments on a draft of the manuscript.

Conflicts of Interest: T.K. reports personal compensation from Biogen Japan and Novartis Japan, and grant support from Novartis Japan. S.I. reports grant support from Novartis Japan. H.A. reports personal compensation from Biogen Japan and Novartis Japan, and grant support from Novartis Japan. H.S. (Hideki Shimomura) reports personal compensation from Biogen Japan. T.S. reports personal compensation from Biogen Japan. T.H. reports personal compensation from Biogen Japan and Novartis Japan. K.S. reports personal compensation from Biogen Japan, Novartis Japan and Chugai Pharmaceutical Co. and grant support from Biogen Japan and Novartis Japan. H.S. (Haruo Shintaku) reports personal compensation from Biogen Japan. K.N. reports grant support from Novartis Japan. Y.T. reports personal compensation from Biogen Japan and Novartis Japan, and grant support from Novartis Japan, and consulting fee from Chugai Pharmaceutical Co. K.I. reports grant support from Novartis Japan. H.N. reports personal compensation from Biogen Japan, Novartis Japan, and Chugai Pharmaceutical Co., and a consulting fee from Sekisui Medical Co. M.S. reports personal compensation and grant support from Biogen Japan. The companies had no role in the design, execution, interpretation, or writing of the study. The other co-authors declare no competing interests.

References

1. Nurputra, D.K.; Lai, P.S.; Harahap, N.I.F.; Morikawa, S.; Yamamoto, T.; Nishimura, N.; Kubo, Y.; Takeuchi, A.; Saito, T.; Takeshima, Y.; et al. Spinal Muscular Atrophy: From Gene Discovery to Clinical Trials. *Ann. Hum. Genet.* **2013**, *77*, 435–463. [CrossRef] [PubMed]
2. Verhaart, I.E.C.; Robertson, A.; Wilson, I.J.; Aartsma-Rus, A.; Cameron, S.; Jones, C.C.; Cook, S.F.; Lochmüller, H. Prevalence, Incidence and Carrier Frequency of 5q-Linked Spinal Muscular Atrophy—A Literature Review. *Orphanet J. Rare Dis.* **2017**, *12*, 124. [CrossRef]
3. Lefebvre, S.; Bürglen, L.; Reboullet, S.; Clermont, O.; Burlet, P.; Viollet, L.; Benichou, B.; Cruaud, C.; Millasseau, P.; Zeviani, M.; et al. Identification and Characterization of a Spinal Muscular Atrophy-Determining Gene. *Cell* **1995**, *80*, 155–165. [CrossRef]
4. Calucho, M.; Bernal, S.; Alías, L.; March, F.; Venceslá, A.; Rodríguez-Álvarez, F.J.; Aller, E.; Fernández, R.M.; Borrego, S.; Millán, J.M.; et al. Correlation between SMA Type and *SMN2* Copy Number Revisited: An Analysis of 625 Unrelated Spanish Patients and a Compilation of 2834 Reported Cases. *Neuromuscul. Disord.* **2018**, *28*, 208–215. [CrossRef] [PubMed]
5. Arnold, W.D.; Kassar, D.; Kissel, J.T. Spinal Muscular Atrophy: Diagnosis and Management in a New Therapeutic Era. *Muscle Nerve* **2015**, *51*, 157–167. [CrossRef]
6. Lally, C.; Jones, C.; Farwell, W.; Reyna, S.P.; Cook, S.F.; Flanders, W.D. Indirect Estimation of the Prevalence of Spinal Muscular Atrophy Type I, II, and III in the United States. *Orphanet J. Rare Dis.* **2017**, *12*, 175. [CrossRef]
7. Oskoui, M.; Levy, G.; Garland, C.J.; Gray, J.M.; O'Hagen, J.; De Vivo, D.C.; Kaufmann, P. The Changing Natural History of Spinal Muscular Atrophy Type 1. *Neurology* **2007**, *69*, 1931–1936. [CrossRef] [PubMed]
8. Neil, E.E.; Bisaccia, E.K. Nusinersen: A Novel Antisense Oligonucleotide for the Treatment of Spinal Muscular Atrophy. *J. Pediatr. Pharmacol. Ther.* **2019**, *24*, 194–203. [CrossRef]
9. Stevens, D.; Claborn, M.K.; Gildon, B.L.; Kessler, T.L.; Walker, C. Onasemnogene Abeparvovec-Xioi: Gene Therapy for Spinal Muscular Atrophy. *Ann. Pharmacother.* **2020**, *54*, 1001–1009. [CrossRef]
10. Finkel, R.S.; Mercuri, E.; Darras, B.T.; Connolly, A.M.; Kuntz, N.L.; Kirschner, J.; Chiriboga, C.A.; Saito, K.; Servais, L.; Tizzano, E.; et al. Nusinersen versus Sham Control in Infantile-Onset Spinal Muscular Atrophy. *N. Engl. J. Med.* **2017**, *377*, 1723–1732. [CrossRef]
11. Mendell, J.R.; Al-Zaidy, S.; Shell, R.; Arnold, W.D.; Rodino-Klapac, L.R.; Prior, T.W.; Lowes, L.; Alfano, L.; Berry, K.; Church, K.; et al. Single-Dose Gene-Replacement Therapy for Spinal Muscular Atrophy. *N. Engl. J. Med.* **2017**, *377*, 1713–1722. [CrossRef] [PubMed]
12. De Vivo, D.C.; Bertini, E.; Swoboda, K.J.; Hwu, W.L.; Crawford, T.O.; Finkel, R.S.; Kirschner, J.; Kuntz, N.L.; Parsons, J.A.; Ryan, M.M.; et al. Nusinersen Initiated in Infants during the Presymptomatic Stage of Spinal Muscular Atrophy: Interim Efficacy and Safety Results from the Phase 2 NURTURE Study. *Neuromuscul. Disord.* **2019**, *29*, 842–856. [CrossRef]
13. Lowes, L.P.; Alfano, L.N.; Arnold, W.D.; Shell, R.; Prior, T.W.; McColly, M.; Lehman, K.J.; Church, K.; Sproule, D.M.; Nagendran, S.; et al. Impact of Age and Motor Function in a Phase 1/2A Study of Infants With SMA Type 1 Receiving Single-Dose Gene Replacement Therapy. *Pediatr. Neurol.* **2019**, *98*, 39–45. [CrossRef] [PubMed]
14. Dangouloff, T.; Vrščaj, E.; Servais, L.; Osredkar, D.; SMA NBS World Study Group. Newborn screening programs for spinal muscular atrophy worldwide: Where we stand and where to go. *Neuromuscul Disord.* **2021**, *31*, 574–582. [CrossRef]
15. Van der Steege, G. PCR-based DNA test to confirm clinical diagnosis of autosomal recessive spinal muscular atrophy. *Lancet* **1995**, *345*, 985–986. [CrossRef]
16. Arkblad, E.L.; Darin, N.; Berg, K.; Kimber, E.; Brandberg, G.; Lindberg, C.; Holmberg, E.; Tulinius, M.; Nordling, M. Multiplex ligation-dependent probe amplification improves diagnostics in spinal muscular atrophy. *Neuromuscul Disord.* **2006**, *16*, 830–838. [CrossRef]

17. Harada, Y.; Sutomo, R.; Sadewa, A.H.; Akutsu, T.; Takeshima, Y.; Wada, H.; Matsuo, M.; Nishio, H. Correlation between *SMN2* copy number and clinical phenotype of spinal muscular atrophy: Three *SMN2* copies fail to rescue some patients from the disease severity. *J. Neurol.* **2002**, *249*, 1211–1219. [CrossRef]
18. Tran, V.K.; Sasongko, T.H.; Hong, D.D.; Hoan, N.T.; Dung, V.C.; Lee, M.J.; Gunadi; Takeshima, Y.; Matsuo, M.; Nishio, H. SMN2 and NAIP Gene Dosages in Vietnamese Patients with Spinal Muscular Atrophy. *Pediatr. Int.* **2008**, *50*, 346–351. [CrossRef] [PubMed]
19. Taylor, J.L.; Lee, F.K.; Yazdanpanah, G.K.; Staropoli, J.F.; Liu, M.; Carulli, J.P.; Sun, C.; Dobrowolski, S.F.; Hannon, W.H.; Vogt, R.F. Newborn blood spot screening test using multiplexed real-time PCR to simultaneously screen for spinal muscular atrophy and severe combined immunodeficiency. *Clin. Chem.* **2015**, *61*, 412–419. [CrossRef] [PubMed]
20. Karakaya, M.; Storbeck, M.; Strathmann, E.A.; Delle Vedove, A.; Hölker, I.; Altmueller, J.; Naghiyeva, L.; Schmitz-Steinkrüger, L.; Vezyroglou, K.; Motameny, S.; et al. Targeted Sequencing with Expanded Gene Profile Enables High Diagnostic Yield in Non-5q-Spinal Muscular Atrophies. *Hum. Mutat.* **2018**, *39*, 1284–1298. [CrossRef] [PubMed]
21. Hosokawa, S.; Kubo, Y.; Arakawa, R.; Takashima, H.; Saito, K. Analysis of spinal muscular atrophy-like patients by targeted resequencing. *Brain Dev.* **2020**, *42*, 148–156. [CrossRef] [PubMed]
22. Wijaya, Y.O.S.; Ar Rochmah, M.; Niba, E.T.E.; Morisada, N.; Noguchi, Y.; Hidaka, Y.; Ozasa, S.; Inoue, T.; Shimazu, T.; Takahashi, Y.; et al. Phenotypes of SMA Patients Retaining *SMN1* with Intragenic Mutation. *Brain Dev.* **2021**, *43*, 745–758. [CrossRef]
23. Yamamoto, T.; Sato, H.; Lai, P.S.; Nurputra, D.K.; Harahap, N.I.F.; Morikawa, S.; Nishimura, N.; Kurashige, T.; Ohshita, T.; Nakajima, H.; et al. Intragenic Mutations in *SMN1* May Contribute More Significantly to Clinical Severity than *SMN2* Copy Numbers in Some Spinal Muscular Atrophy (SMA) Patients. *Brain Dev.* **2014**, *36*, 914–920. [CrossRef]
24. Wirth, B.; Herz, M.; Wetter, A.; Moskau, S.; Hahnen, E.; Rudnik-Schöneborn, S.; Wienker, T.; Zerres, K. Quantitative Analysis of Survival Motor Neuron Copies: Identification of Subtle *SMN1* Mutations in Patients with Spinal Muscular Atrophy, Genotype-Phenotype Correlation, and Implications for Genetic Counseling. *Am. J. Hum. Genet.* **1999**, *64*, 1340–1356. [CrossRef]
25. Al-Jumah, M.; Majumdar, R.; Al-Rajeh, S.; Awada, A.; Chaves-Carballo, E.; Salih, M.; Al-Shahwan, S.; Al-Subiey, K.; Al-Uthaim, S. Molecular Analysis of the Spinal Muscular Atrophy and Neuronal Apoptosis Inhibitory Protein Genes in Saudi Patients with Spinal Muscular Atrophy. *Saudi Med. J.* **2003**, *24*, 1052–1054. [PubMed]
26. Labrum, R.; Rodda, J.; Krause, A. The Molecular Basis of Spinal Muscular Atrophy (SMA) in South African Black Patients. *Neuromuscul. Disord.* **2007**, *17*, 684–692. [CrossRef]
27. Watihayati, M.S.; Zabidi-Hussin, A.M.H.; Tang, T.H.; Nishio, H.; Zilfalil, B.A. NAIP-Deletion Analysis in Malaysian Patients with Spinal Muscular Atrophy. *Kobe J. Med. Sci.* **2007**, *53*, 171–175.
28. Belter, L.; Cook, S.F.; Crawford, T.O.; Jarecki, J.; Jones, C.C.; Kissel, J.T.; Schroth, M.; Hobby, K. An Overview of the Cure SMA Membership Database: Highlights of Key Demographic and Clinical Characteristics of SMA Members. *J. Neuromuscul. Dis.* **2018**, *5*, 167–176. [CrossRef] [PubMed]
29. Okamoto, K.; Fukuda, M.; Saito, I.; Urate, R.; Maniwa, S.; Usui, D.; Motoki, T.; Jogamoto, T.; Aibara, K.; Hosokawa, T.; et al. Incidence of Infantile Spinal Muscular Atrophy on Shikoku Island of Japan. *Brain Dev.* **2019**, *41*, 36–42. [CrossRef]
30. Sun, Y.; Kong, X.; Zhao, Z.; Zhao, X. Mutation Analysis of 419 Family and Prenatal Diagnosis of 339 Cases of Spinal Muscular Atrophy in China. *BMC Med. Genet.* **2020**, *21*, 133. [CrossRef] [PubMed]
31. Kekou, K.; Svingou, M.; Sofocleous, C.; Mourtzi, N.; Nitsa, E.; Konstantinidis, G.; Youroukos, S.; Skiadas, K.; Katsalouli, M.; Pons, R.; et al. Evaluation of Genotypes and Epidemiology of Spinal Muscular Atrophy in Greece: A Nationwide Study Spanning 24 Years. *J. Neuromuscul. Dis.* **2020**, *7*, 247–256. [CrossRef]
32. Lin, C.W.; Kalb, S.J.; Yeh, W.S. Delay in Diagnosis of Spinal Muscular Atrophy: A Systematic Literature Review. *Pediatr. Neurol.* **2015**, *53*, 293–300. [CrossRef]
33. Pera, M.C.; Coratti, G.; Berti, B.; D'Amico, A.; Sframeli, M.; Albamonte, E.; De Sanctis, R.; Messina, S.; Catteruccia, M.; Brigati, G.; et al. Diagnostic Journey in Spinal Muscular Atrophy: Is It Still an Odyssey? *PLoS ONE.* **2020**, *15*, e0230677. [CrossRef]
34. Imaizumi, Y. Incidence and Mortality Rates of Werdnig-Hoffmann Disease in Japan, 1979–1996. *Hyogo Univ. Arch.* **1996**, *13*, 53–59.
35. Arkblad, E.; Tulinius, M.; Kroksmark, A.K.; Henricsson, M.; Darin, N. A Population-Based Study of Genotypic and Phenotypic Variability in Children with Spinal Muscular Atrophy. *Acta Paediatr. Int. J. Paediatr.* **2009**, *98*, 865–872. [CrossRef] [PubMed]
36. Jedrzejowska, M.; Milewski, M.; Zimowski, J.; Zagozdzon, P.; Kostera-Pruszczyk, A.; Borkowska, J.; Sielska, D.; Jurek, M.; Hausmanowa-Petrusewicz, I. Incidence of Spinal Muscular Atrophy in Poland—More Frequent than Predicted? *Neuroepidemiology* **2010**, *34*, 152–157. [CrossRef] [PubMed]
37. Vaidla, E.; Talvik, I.; Kulla, A.; Kahre, T.; Hamarik, M.; Napa, A.; Metsvaht, T.; Piirsoo, A.; Talvik, T. Descriptive Epidemiology of Spinal Muscular Atrophy Type I in Estonia. *Neuroepidemiology* **2006**, *27*, 164–168. [CrossRef]
38. Prior, T.W.; Snyder, P.J.; Rink, B.D.; Pearl, D.K.; Pyatt, R.E.; Mihal, D.C.; Conlan, T.; Schmalz, B.; Montgomery, L.; Ziegler, K.; et al. Newborn and Carrier Screening for Spinal Muscular Atrophy. *Am. J. Med. Genet. A* **2010**, *152A*, 1608–1616. [CrossRef] [PubMed]
39. Chien, Y.H.; Chiang, S.C.; Weng, W.C.; Lee, N.C.; Lin, C.J.; Hsieh, W.S.; Lee, W.T.; Jong, Y.J.; Ko, T.M.; Hwu, W.L. Presymptomatic Diagnosis of Spinal Muscular Atrophy Through Newborn Screening. *J. Pediatr.* **2017**, *190*, 124–129.e1. [CrossRef] [PubMed]
40. Kraszewski, J.N.; Kay, D.M.; Stevens, C.F.; Koval, C.; Haser, B.; Ortiz, V.; Albertorio, A.; Cohen, L.L.; Jain, R.; Andrew, S.P.; et al. Pilot Study of Population-Based Newborn Screening for Spinal Muscular Atrophy in New York State. *Genet. Med.* **2018**, *20*, 608–613. [CrossRef]

41. Shinohara, M.; Niba, E.T.E.; Wijaya, Y.O.S.; Takayama, I.; Mitsuishi, C.; Kumasaka, S.; Kondo, Y.; Takatera, A.; Hokuto, I.; Morioka, I.; et al. A Novel System for Spinal Muscular Atrophy Screening in Newborns: Japanese Pilot Study Masakazu. *Int. J. Neonatal Screen.* **2019**, *5*, 41. [CrossRef]
42. Vill, K.; Schwartz, O.; Blaschek, A.; Gläser, D.; Nennstiel, U.; Wirth, B.; Burggraf, S.; Röschinger, W.; Becker, M.; Czibere, L.; et al. Newborn Screening for Spinal Muscular Atrophy in Germany: Clinical Results after 2 Years. *Orphanet J. Rare Dis.* **2021**, *16*, 153. [CrossRef]
43. Kariyawasam, D.S.T.; D'Silva, A.M.; Vetsch, J.; Wakefield, C.E.; Wiley, V.; Farrar, M.A. "We Needed This": Perspectives of Parents and Healthcare Professionals Involved in a Pilot Newborn Screening Program for Spinal Muscular Atrophy. *EClinicalMedicine* **2021**, *33*, 1–11. [CrossRef]
44. Kucera, K.S.; Taylor, J.L.; Robles, V.R.; Clinard, K.; Migliore, B.; Boyea, B.L.; Okoniewski, K.C.; Duparc, M.; Rehder, C.W.; Shone, S.M.; et al. A Voluntary Statewide Newborn Screening Pilot for Spinal Muscular Atrophy: Results from Early Check. *Int. J. Neonatal Screen.* **2021**, *7*, 20. [CrossRef]
45. Harahap, N.I.F.; Harahap, I.S.K.; Kaszynski, R.H.; Nurputra, D.K.P.; Hartomo, T.B.; Pham, H.T.V.; Yamamoto, T.; Morikawa, S.; Nishimura, N.; Rusdi, I.; et al. Spinal Muscular Atrophy Patient Detection and Carrier Screening Using Dried Blood Spots on Filter Paper. *Genet. Test. Mol. Biomarkers* **2012**, *16*, 123–129. [CrossRef] [PubMed]
46. Sa'adah, N.; Harahap, N.I.F.; Nurputra, D.K.P.; Ar Rochmah, M.; Morikawa, S.; Nishimura, N.; Sadewa, A.H.; Astuti, I.; Haryana, S.M.; Saito, T.; et al. A Rapid, Accurate and Simple Screening Method for Spinal Muscular Atrophy: High-Resolution Melting Analysis Using Dried Blood Spots on Filter Paper. *Clin. Lab.* **2015**, *61*, 575–580. [CrossRef] [PubMed]
47. Wijaya, Y.O.S.; Purevsuren, J.; Harahap, N.I.F.; Niba, E.T.E.; Bouike, Y.; Nurputra, D.K.P.; Ar Rochmah, M.; Thursina, C.; Hapsara, S.; Yamaguchi, S.; et al. Assessment of Spinal Muscular Atrophy Carrier Status by Determining *SMN1* Copy Number Using Dried Blood Spots. *Int. J. Neonatal Screen.* **2020**, *6*, 43. [CrossRef] [PubMed]
48. Japanese Researchers Develop Neonatal SMA Test to Start Treatment before Symptoms—June 18, 2021 (Mainichi Japan). Available online: https://web.archive.org/web/20210628022802/https://mainichi.jp/english/articles/20210617/p2a/00m/0na/015000c (accessed on 28 June 2021).

MDPI\
St. Alban-Anlage 66\
4052 Basel\
Switzerland\
Tel. +41 61 683 77 34\
Fax +41 61 302 89 18\
www.mdpi.com

International Journal of Neonatal Screening Editorial Office\
E-mail: ijns@mdpi.com\
www.mdpi.com/journal/ijns

www.ingramcontent.com/pod-product-compliance
Lightning Source LLC
LaVergne TN
LVHW070043120526
838202LV00101B/417